# Occupational Therapy and Inclusive Design: Principles for Practice

# Occupational Therapy and Inclusive Design: Principles for Practice

Maggie Conway

Illustrations by Kasia Halota

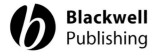
Blackwell
Publishing

Blackwell Publishing was acquired by John Wiley & Sons in February 2007. Blackwell's publishing programme has been merged with Wiley's global Scientific, Technical, and Medical business to form Wiley-Blackwell.

*Registered office*
John Wiley & Sons Ltd, The Atrium, Southern Gate, Chichester, West Sussex, PO19 8SQ, United Kingdom

*Editorial office*
9600 Garsington Road, Oxford, OX4 2DQ, United Kingdom

For details of our global editorial offices, for customer services and for information about how to apply for permission to reuse the copyright material in this book please see our website at www.wiley.com/wiley-blackwell.

*Library of Congress Cataloging-in-Publication Data*
Conway, Maggie.
Occupational therapy and inclusive design : principles for practice / Maggie Conway.
p. ; cm.
Includes bibliographical references and index.
ISBN-13: 978-1-4051-2707-3 (pbk. : alk. paper)
ISBN-10: 1-4051-2707-4 (pbk. : alk. paper)    1. Occupational therapy.    2. People with disabilities.    3. Universal design.    4. Barrier-free design.    5. Engineering design.    I. Title.
[DNLM:    1. Occupational Therapy–psychology.    2. Models, Psychological. WB 555 C767o 2008]

RM735.C668 2008
615.8′515–dc22
2007039649

A catalogue record for this book is available from the British Library.

Set in 10 on 12.5 pt Palatino by SNP Best-set Typesetter Ltd., Hong Kong
Printed in Singapore by C. O. S. Printers Pte Ltd

1   2008

Dedication

With grateful thanks and much love.

To my parents Gretta and Thomas whose early guidance
developed the resolve.

To my husband Giovanni Zammit whose unwavering support, optimism and
timely cups of tea, saw this work safely through.

To my children, Matthew and Jack, who understood why mum was busy and
so boring.

# Contents

# Acknowledgements

The author gratefully acknowledges the following for their help and support during the development and completion of this book.

Katrina Chandler, Commissioning Editor of the Health Science, Addiction and Dentistry Division, and Amy Brown, Managing Editor of the Professional Division, both at Blackwell Publishing, whose support and encouragement were readily available during all stages of the writing.

Erik Koornneef, Senior Standards Officer, National Disability Authority, Dublin, Ireland (www.nda.ie), for permission to use images in Chapter 8. The use of these images greatly supports and illuminates this section.

Mary Morley, Director of Therapies at South West London and St George's Mental Health NHS Trust, for encouragement during all stages of the process and for the use of her apartment as a writer's den during a time of much-needed solitude.

Kasia Halota, whose wonderful illustrations enliven the text.

John Conway, whose timely solution to a scanning problem saved the day.

Grateful thanks are due to all.

# Introduction

The purpose of this publication is to explore the interdisciplinary knowledge base needed to promote satisfying and effective occupational performance for all, but particularly with regard to a discrete group – disabled people. Occupational performance may be described as:

> 'The result of a dynamic, interwoven relationship between persons, environment, and occupation over a person's lifespan; the ability to choose, organise, and satisfactorily perform meaningful occupations that are culturally defined and age appropriate for looking after oneself, enjoying life, and contributing to the social and economic fabric of a community' (CAOT 1997, p.181).

Occupational therapists and others involved in the design and development of environments for use by disabled people must continually keep abreast of and contribute to evolving perceptions relating to an understanding of disability and how this is conceptualised. Practitioners and other stakeholders should understand how our beliefs and attitudes influence and shape the occupational performance experience, for good or ill, of the many disabled people in our communities.

Inclusive design (also referred to as universal design), a design concept that aims to embrace the diversity of human ability, challenges the traditional design notion that designing for disabled users as part of the total user population will lead to inferior design practice (Orstroff 2001).

Occupational therapists can become key players in the advocacy and use of this approach within their practice and through using the guiding principles of the inclusive or universal design process can develop a set of skills, knowledge and evidence to underpin practice, working towards meeting service users' needs and thereby promoting greater inclusion and participation, and ultimately enhancing the occupational performance satisfaction of disabled people. More importantly, practitioners can mount a challenge to the disenfranchisement of disabled people and advocate for their rights as equal citizens to fully participate in, shape and enrich our future society.

The first part of this publication considers the development and evolution of disability perspectives through history to the present day. An overview of disability discourse through the ages, from the Middle Ages through the Early Modern period (18th and 19th centuries) up to the 20th century and beyond will be presented and critically considered. The views we hold about 'difference' – for the purposes of this publication, those that relate to disability – have developed over generations and have slowly and steadily become part of our consciousness and shaped our perceptions. In order to be able to truly embrace the disability movement cause and adopt the social model of disability as a primary influence, we must first understand – at least to some degree – why we hold the perceptions we do.

The disability models and discourses that influence and shape our understanding of disability and that determine society's perception of disability will be critically reviewed and related to the dominant models of service provision within health and social care but also within society more broadly. It is hoped that a review of the discourses that have shaped society's relationship with and consequently our perceptions of disabled people may go some way towards deepening our understanding of the root causes of handicap – the experience of being prevented from participating as an equal player. Our changing perceptions and challenges from the disability rights movements have led to the present-day need to review and reframe our understanding of this relationship.

Occupational therapy (OT) perspectives are not static; they are dynamic and so are continually evolving within the ever-changing sociopolitical, sociocultural, biopsychosocial and technical contexts within which our practice is situated.

Through a firm understanding of the occupational performance needs of our clients, occupational therapists are already well placed to integrate the principles of inclusive or universal design with the profession's core beliefs. Universal design aims to promote the development of a design concept that simplifies life for everyone, able-bodied and disabled alike, by making our built environments, artefacts and communications more accessible to a range of users without increased cost implications (Mace 1997).

The concept is supported by seven principles and focuses on all design disciplines relating to the environment (built and social), products/artefacts and communications. These principles and their application to practice will be addressed in Part 2. The need for OTs to have a sound understanding of ergonomic principles will be explored and related to practice. Case scenarios will be presented. Application of the principles of universal design to practice will be considered within the context of equipment specification and built environment recommendations. Applications will address the physical, psychosocial and cognitive needs of clients/service users and will be explored with good practice examples presented. The principles of inclusive design, a term used more commonly in the UK and European contexts, are the dominant focus of this publication. It tends to encompass a broader understanding to include the design of mechanisms to help reduce attitudinal and social barriers.

Part 3 of this book will critically consider legislative and policy developments within the UK and elsewhere and how these impact on practice. It will ask the question 'Do policy and the law go far enough?'. The response of the World Health Organization (WHO) to the disability movement will be critically considered in the light of the shift from a purely medical classification of illness and impairment (ICD) to a classification more fitting to the needs of the disabled community; a classification that acknowledges that disability does not automatically equate with illness; a classification that acknowledges that the elements of 'activity and participation' are key indicators in determining quality of life levels for the disabled community. These indicators are more meaningful for disabled people and shift the focus from the disabled individual (medical model perspective) to the obligations of society (social model perspective).

Other national legislation, guidance and policies such as the NHS Plan 2000, National Service Frameworks, MHOR 1992, PUWER 1998 and LOLER 1998 will also be presented and considered as a means to equip and inform practitioners in their goal to implement best practice.

This section will also present a global perspective on disability through reviewing and critically considering a range of international legislative and policy frameworks such as the United Nations Standard Rules for the Equalization of Opportunity for Persons with Disabilities, UK, France, Germany, Italy, The Netherlands, USA, Canada, Australia.

Essentially this book aims to explore the relationship between our perspectives and attitudes concerning disability and how these perspectives have shaped the lived experience of disabled people; for many it is a lived experience of marginalisation and social exclusion; of being judged as 'so different' from the able-bodied community as to justify different treatment and lower expectations. Such attitudes have been a key factor in the development and organisation of societal and legislative structures that prevent the participation of disabled people as equal players in society. Handicapped by society and not by disability is the result. The principles that guide the universal design and inclusive design perspectives will help to open our eyes and show us a better way towards a, potentially, truly inclusive world. This approach goes further than many of the grand theories and ideologies that relate to inclusion – inclusive and universal design gives us the road map.

## References

Canadian Association of Occupational Therapists (CAOT) (1997) *Enabling Occupation: an occupational therapy perspective*. CAOT Publications, Ottawa, Canada.

Mace R (1997) *The Principles of Universal Design (Version 2.0)*. Center for Universal Design, North Carolina State University, Raleigh, North Carolina.

Ostroff E (2001) Universal design: the new paradigm. In: Preiser W, Ostroff E (eds) *Universal Design Handbook*. McGraw-Hill, New York.

# PART 1
# The Sociocultural and Professional Context

'The significance of a disability always depends on more than its biological nature, it is shaped by the human circumstances in which it exists' (Ingstad and Whyte 1995).

# 1: Cultural production of disability

This chapter aims to provide an overview of the disability discourses down the ages from ancient times to the present day and to present to the reader the subtle influences that have shaped our perspectives on disability. Perhaps we may feel that our view of disabled people is entirely laudable and that we have a good understanding of the lived experience of disabled people and so may feel that this section is not relevant. The reader must be the judge of such issues and indeed, this book allows the reader to dip into and out of topics as desired. The beliefs we hold, however, are not accidental nor incidental but have been inserted into our consciousnesses, steadily over many generations, and have been reinforced in the nursery rhymes we learned as children, through the literature we have read and by the films we watched. To understand something of this process and perhaps to consider that we may indeed be more tainted than we know, we must first look back and unlearn and only then, equipped with greater understanding, move forward.

This section aims to acquaint the reader with some of the possible subtle influences that may be buried in our subconscious and which form part of the contemporary collective subconscious. The views that govern our responses to disability, and indeed to all phenomena that are perceived as being in some way different from the norm, have taken root in the past and, depending on how these phenomena were understood by our forebears, determine largely the present perceptions that have been generated with regard to 'difference'. For the purpose of this text the 'difference' we are concerned with is that of disability and the disabled in our society today.

Perceptions do not merely 'happen' or 'appear' suddenly but are the result of subtle processes of understanding, the formulation and reformulation of hypotheses, the development of paradigms, theories and models and the acceptance as 'true' of opinions presented by the 'experts' on a given subject.

To better understand the evolutionary knowledge base that underpins our understanding of disability, readers need to look to the past, both their own and society's, for some clues that may solve or at least provide some insights into the conundrum.

## Fairies and the folklore of disability: changelings, hybrids and the solitary fairy

Therefore the author makes no apology for opening the first section of this text with a review of early folklore, of the customs and traditions that shaped the cultural perspective of the time and that undoubtedly shaped the early views of disability and that to some extent continue to exert an influence today. It is likely that our present interpretation and understanding of disability are influenced by this legacy.

Young (1997) suggests that myths and legends are common to every society, culture and country and that the fairy stories and folk tales of our ancestors form part of our collective consciousness and subconscious thought. To some degree our present understanding, at both the individual and societal levels, of personal issues and social values continues to be shaped by their influence and so a brief review of folklore and historical perspective concerning the disability worldviews may illuminate the contemporary perspective.

In the absence of a clear evidence-based understanding of disability and other inexplicable life events, a system or paradigm of fairy belief arose and provided one way in which life's more mysterious events and occurrences could be understood (Frazer 1971). Events such as the untimely death of young people, mysterious epidemics among cattle, climatic disaster, wasting diseases and strokes, infantile paralysis and the birth of 'Mongol' or otherwise 'different' children required an explanation, an explanation that provided an answer for the particular community. Answers that were acceptable to the community were those that posed no threat to its members. In the case of disability the 'different' individuals, it is thought (Schoon-Eberly 1988), were ascribed the title of *chretien* (Christian) as it was believed that they were God's children. It was believed that God's wrath had fallen on such individuals and thus the community in which this person lived would not be visited by God's anger again. It is suggested that the term 'cretin' may have derived from this origin (Schoon-Eberly 1988). Braddock and Parish (2001) note that infants with sensory impairments or those with a learning disability were not routinely identified as 'deformed' at birth and so were not put to death. It is likely that their impairments were not discovered until early childhood and that they were then past the age when it would be considered appropriate to put the child to death by exposure.

Children born with major physical defects have evoked a religious response since at least as early as 2000 BC. It was believed that such births would lead to disaster for the community: 'the country will be in affliction, the house will be destroyed, the town will have no births' (Schoon-Eberly 1988, p.58). In Rome at that time children with visible defects were particularly valued for sacrifice in times of emergency. The belief that there was a link between the supernatural and deformed children persisted through the Middle Ages and into the Reformation and beyond. It persists in some cultures of the world even in modern times. Ingstad (1997) cites from her work *Community-based Rehabilitation in Botswana* the following:

> 'Disability seen as a Divine curse justifies low self esteem for disabled people and their families . . . Moral trespasses or "sins" and "evil thoughts" may remain hidden, but the appearance of a disability in a family will make the "sin" visible to all' (p.84).

Ingstad and Whyte (1995) note that in the case of unexplained impairment, anger and denial also tend to be part of the corresponding reaction. Such reactions tend to be bound up not only with fear of the unknown but also with the desire for sameness.

It is reasonable to assume that primitive societies both ancient and modern needed the active contribution of all their members to ensure the survival of the community. It is likely that caring for the infirm in the more primitive societies places an unwanted burden on the particular family and community concerned.

Colridge (1993) states that disability is primarily a social problem because what prevents the individual disabled person from contributing is the attitude of the non-disabled person towards him or her and not the disability per se.

Folklore and superstition the world over have incorporated into their essence the plight of those individuals afflicted with a visible disability or whose behaviour is judged 'different' and is in some way 'lesser' and so to be pitied or despised by the tribe.

## The changeling

Schoon-Eberly (1988) suggests that the emergence of the 'changeling' tales represents an aspect of the parents' grieving process, the rejection of the disabled child and the sense of loss for the 'wished-for' baby. These feelings continue to change as part of the grieving process and over time give way to feelings of denial, guilt and sometimes anger.

In reference to Lewis Spence's work *The Fairy Traditions in Britain*, Schoon-Eberly (1988) discusses the role of the fairy changeling. She notes that wherever a cretinous or diseased child made its appearance in a family, it was usually regarded as a changeling and that the individual case was made to fit the superstition, and thus we possess no standardised data representing the appearance of a changeling. The 'changeling' was believed to be a fairy child which was substituted for a healthy human baby. The 'changeling' was often sickly and mute, and deformed in some way. The human baby it was believed to have replaced was stolen by the fairies.

The following tale is reported of a family in Cornwall.

> 'There was a fine baby girl . . . and the piskies came and took it and put a withered child in its place. The withered child lived to be 20 years old . . . It was fretful and peevish and frightfully shrivelled' (Schoon-Eberly 1988, p.61).

The concept of 'fairy races' may in fact have been generated in response to the physical similarities manifest by certain medical syndromes. Williams syndrome or hypercalcaemia also goes by the name of 'elfin facies' syndrome. Unusual ears, perhaps large and differently shaped, and 'mongoloid' eyes, having epicanthic folds, tend to be trademark features of many fairy illustrations; these features are also common to many medical syndromes, of which Down's syndrome is a familiar example. Some others are presented below.

The rare syndrome progeria is the result of a metabolic disorder and those affected will never grow to be larger than a five-year-old. The condition is essentially the acceleration of the ageing process. It is possible that the tale of 'Yallery Brown' draws on this syndrome for inspiration. 'Yallery Brown, tiny but ancient looking, with his fine hair and his brown skin, his face as wrinkled and as brown as the earth' (Schoon-Eberly 1988, p.70). 'Yallery Brown' tells of a child left to die under a stone by his parents, the belief being that the fey folk would not allow one of their own to perish and that the 'changeling' would be rescued by them and the human child returned. The physical description of Yallery Brown is consistent with that of a child with progeria.

Other conditions worthy of mention include metabolic disorders such as phenylketonuria (PKU) and homocystinuria. In PKU, those affected are often fair-skinned with blond hair and blue eyes even when the parents are not; they will have an overall small body form and, if left untreated, will have severe learning disability. Microcephaly sometimes occurs and cerebral palsy develops in about one-third of all cases. In homocystinuria, osteoporosis, learning disability and cerebral palsy are also present in the majority of cases. Arachnodactyly is common to this syndrome; this refers to limbs and digits which are extremely long and thin or 'spider-like'. Those with PKU tend to be elfin or pixie-like in appearance whilst those with homocystinuria tend to have a more generalised fairy appearance.

The fate of some of these 'changelings' was monstrous and amounted to little more than socially countenanced forms of infanticide. Martin Luther labelled one severely retarded child as a 'massa carnis' (soulless mass of flesh) (Schoon-Eberly 1988, p.60) and recommended that the child be disposed of by drowning. Others were 'thrown on a bed of glowing coals or left below the high-water mark when the tide was out' (Schoon-Eberly 1988, pp.61–62).

## Hybrids

Folklore includes tales of creatures that have been produced from human and non-human or supernatural mating, such as with gods, devils, incubi, succubi, fairies, mermaids, etc. More mundane accounts of hybridity refer to the union of humans and animals although the animals in question often had supernatural associations. The children of such unions generally bore some outward or physical sign of their parentage, such as webbed fingers and toes, scaly skin, cleft pallet, clubfoot. Sirenomelia is one such example and is a congenital condition in which a child is born with fused legs giving the appearance of a 'fish's tail' (Fig. 1.1). Conditions such as these may play some part in the imagery of folklore (Schoon-Eberly 1988).

Syndactyly (webbed digits) is the most common of all congenital malformations. The goat-footed Urisk, a kindly but shy creature half-human and half-fairy, lived in close proximity to humans and helped with the farm chores (Fig. 1.2) (Schoon-Eberly 1988).The inspiration for this character may have been the congenital condition talipes equines in which tip-toe walking is a clinical sign. Indeed, such a gait could also be attributed to a number of other conditions caused by central nervous system damage, including spina bifida and cerebral palsy (Schoon-Eberly1988).

The individual with Marfan's syndrome also presents with a characteristic physical appearance, that may have contributed to beliefs that such individuals were not human. Marfan's syndrome is sometimes called arachnodactyly, which means 'spider-like fingers' in Greek, since one of the characteristic signs of the disease is disproportionately long fingers and toes. It is one of the more common inheritable disorders. The most common external signs associated with Marfan's syndrome include excessively long arms and legs, with the patient's arm span being greater than his or her height. The individual's face may also be long and narrow, and he or she may have a noticeable curvature of the spine (Frey 2002).

## Solitary fairies

Schoon-Eberly (1988) suggests that the 'changelings' who survived infancy are represented in folklore in the tales of the solitary fairies. It

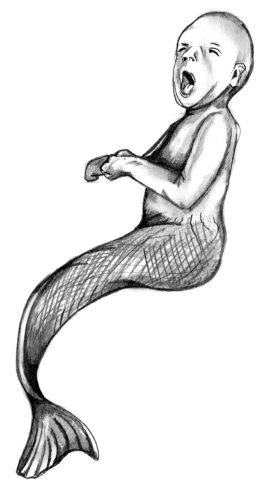

**Figure 1.1** Illustrator's impression of a baby born with sirenomelia. Conditions such as these may play some part in the mermaid imagery of folklore (Schoon-Eberly 1988). (Drawn by Kasia Halota.)

has been suggested that the 'different' child who survives, perhaps with more mental than physical impairment, may also be represented by the 'solitary fairies'. Both the domestic and the more reclusive types, such as the Gille Dubh, Meg Moulach, the Brown Man of the Muirs, the Grogan and the Fenoderree, possessed characteristics which are reminiscent of the person with mental/emotional impairment and/or learning difficulties and were often physically different as well.

The solitary 'nature' fairy who dwelled usually by a well or a stream and hunted, fished or scavenged for survival may well have had one of the syndromes which causes dwarfism. Achondroplastic or short-limbed dwarfism manifests as a trunk of normal size, large head and

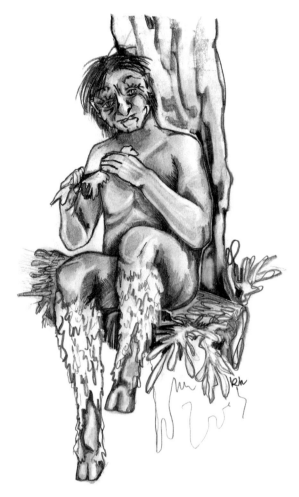

**Figure 1.2** Illustrator's impression of the Urisk. The inspiration for this character may have been the congenital condition talipes equines in which tip-toe walking is a clinical sign (Schoon-Eberly 1988). (Drawn by Kasia Halota.)

very short limbs. Costoverterbral dwarfing results in limbs of normal size, a very short trunk, frequent occurrence of clubfoot and in some cases learning difficulty. Anterior hypopituitary dwarfism, a common dwarfing syndrome, leads to normal body proportions but overall small size.

The mucopolysaccharidosis syndromes should also be considered as a source of inspiration for the images presented in folklore. For instance, those with Hunter's and Hurler's syndromes present with thickset jaws and heavy brows, coarse dark hair covers much of their bodies, the eyes bulge, hands are clawed, they breathe hoarsely, may be humpbacked and are small of stature (Fig. 1.3). Those with Hunter's

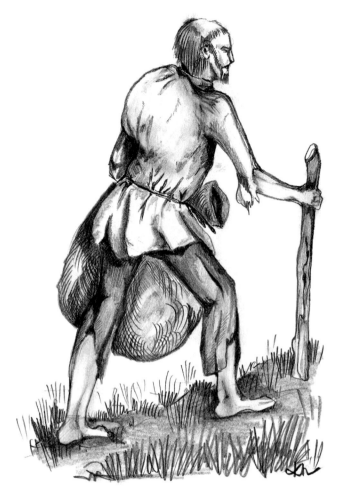

**Figure 1.3** Illustrator's impression of the hunchback from folklore (Schoon-Eberly 1988). (Drawn by Kasia Halota.)

syndrome have a pleasant and loving temperament whilst those with Hurler's are hyperactive, rough, noisy and aggressive. Learning disability is also often present. It is entirely possible that the Brown Man of the Muirs was inspired by an individual with Hurler's syndrome. He is described as a small hideous dwarf, with eyes round and fierce as a bull's, squat, strongly made with an intimidating visage and wild frizzy hair (Fig. 1.4) (Schoon-Eberly 1988).

A 'brownie' is described as short in stature, swarthy, somewhat hairy with coarse, rather unrefined features, nearly always silent and always inhabiting the margins of society (Schoon-Eberly 1988). This description could also be applied to those individuals of the time with

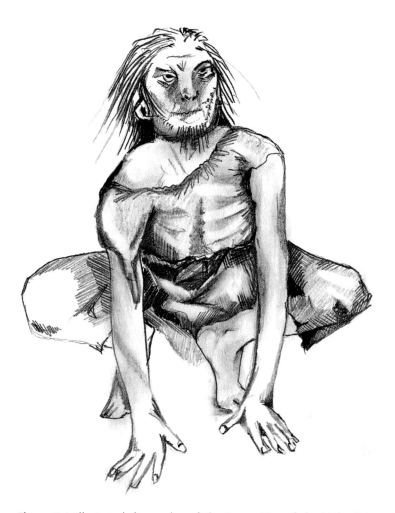

**Figure 1.4** Illustrator's impression of the Brown Man of the Muirs (Schoon-Eberly 1988). (Drawn by Kasia Halota.)

certain cognitive and/or physical disabilities. The medical condition 'cretinism' may have been the inspiration for this creature.

It is likely that the 'brownie' represents 'different' human beings and those people with a learning disability and who also had a physically 'different' appearance and who, because of this, were rejected by a fearful and ignorant society. If not supported by their family – which, as we have seen, was by no means a certainty – they made a meagre living doing the menial tasks required by the community. The experience of these people was one of rejection and exclusion from a fearful community with too few resources (intellectual and material) to support 'different' members.

The Gille Dubh, who lived in the 1800s in Scotland by the edge of Loch During, is described as black-haired, and covered his nakedness with leaves and moss. He was known to be a gentle creature. He could speak but rarely did (Schoon-Eberly1988). The tale tells of a local land-owner's attempts to hunt and capture the Gille Dubh and keep him as a trophy. Such accounts give some insight into the prevailing attitudes towards 'difference', not only physical difference but also behaviour linked to mental illness of some kind. Victimisation, social ostracism and exclusion were prevalent.

This is not an exhaustive list of such conditions and syndromes and many are seen rarely in contemporary Western society. However, the opinions presented here are strong enough to suggest that impairment and deformity were an important inspiration in the images of folklore. The vast majority of these images are negative and it is reasonable to suppose that such images reflected prevailing attitudes of hostility and fear towards those with disabilities (Schoon-Eberly 1988). The evidence suggests that people with disabilities were dealt with harshly by society – they were marginalised and, as has been illustrated, dehumanised.

## References

Braddock D, Parish S (2001) An institutional history of disability. In: Albrecht GL, Seelman KD, Bury M (eds) (2001) *Handbook Of Disability Studies*. Sage Publications, California.

Colridge P (1993) *Disability, Liberation and Development*. Oxfam, London.

Frazer JG (1971) *The Golden Bough: a study in magic and religion* (abridged edn, reprint). Macmillan, Basingstoke.

Frey RJ (2002) *Gale Encyclopedia of Medicine*. Gale Group Publishing, Farmington Hills, Michigan.

Ingstad B (1997) *Community-based Rehabilitation in Botswana: the myth of the hidden disabled*. Edwin Mellen Press, Leviston.

Ingstad B, Reynolds-Whyte S (1995) *Disability and Culture*. University of California Press, Berkeley, California.

Schoon-Eberly S (1988) Fairies and the folklore of disability: changelings, hybrids and the solitary fairy. *Folklore* **99(1)**, 58–77.

Young J (1997) Once upon a time: how fairy tales shape our lives. *Inside Journal* **August**. Available online at: www.folkstory.com/articles/onceupon.

# 2: Disability discourses

The general meaning of the word 'discourse' is dialogue or conversation. It is also used in social theory to describe whole structures of thought within which discussion takes place. Disability, for example, might be described as a discourse or a set of discourses. The idea is that there are structures of thought that are not rigid dogmas, but which guide the thinker and close off options (Foucault 1969). Discourse may be further defined as an understanding of an attitude towards a phenomenon – the phenomenon of interest in this text is that of disability.

A dominant discourse may be described as the spoken, written and behavioural expectations that we all share within a cultural grouping – it becomes the norm. However, because norms are often not part of conscious awareness, they can lead to many unstated assumptions and the generation of stereotypes (Mills 2005). Examples from religion, magic, superstition and primitive culture reflect the harsh treatments by the able-bodied of the disabled in a community. Disability, as we have already noted, was often thought to be the visible manifestation of evil and strange rituals were employed in the exorcising of demons.

The experience of disability is culturally situated and derives from a social construction at a given point in time (Cone 1998). Knowledge is therefore socially constructed in that it evolves through interaction with others (Berger and Luckmann 1996, Gergen 1999, Greene and Lee 2002, Heron and Reason 1997, Laird 1993). Anything we know comes from within a context (Laird 1993). Knowledge is never construed in a void.

Within literature and other forms of cultural representation, discourses of disability and disabled people tend to be one-dimensional, dealing with stereotypes. For example, Barnes (1992) notes that the disabled person is usually (a) a sad pathetic victim, (b) a tragic but brave hero/ine or (c) an evil, twisted villain. Examples from literature illustrate the influence of the earlier folk knowledge and understanding relating to disability and difference.

'But I, that am not shap'd for sportive tricks,
Nor made to court an amorous looking-glass;
I, that am rudely stamp'd, and want love's majesty . . .
I, that am curtail'd of this fair proportion,
Cheated of feature by dissembling natyre,
Deform'd, unfinish'd, sent before my time
Into this breathing world, scarce half made up,
And that so lamely and unfashionable
That dogs bark at me, as I halt by them; . . .
. . . And therefore, since I cannot prove a lover,
To entertain these fair well-spoken days,
I am determined to prove a villain . . .'

This extract, Richard's opening speech from Shakespeare's *The Tragedy of King Richard III*, presents a character as misshapen on the inside as on the exterior. The implicit meaning conveyed suggests that deformity equates with depravity.

## Nursery rhymes

'There was a crooked man, and he went a crooked mile,
He found a crooked sixpence beside a crooked stile;
He bought a crooked cat, which caught a crooked mouse,
And they all lived together in a little crooked house.'

Although this nursery rhyme originates from the English Stuart history of King Charles I, the crooked man is reputed to be the Scottish general Sir Alexander Leslie. The words reflect the time when there was great animosity between the English and the Scots. The image presented is one of disability and exclusion. The origin is unlikely to be known to most children but strong associations with an ageist perspective are presented.

The rhyme below similarly presents a negative view of difference and disability.

'As I was going to sell my eggs,
I met a man with bandy legs,
Bandy legs and crooked toes;
I tripped up his heels,
and he fell on his nose.'

Disability as a social construct was not categorised until the 1700s (Braddock and Parish 2001) yet impairments were commonplace long before then. The response of a particular society at a given time to impaired individuals was largely concerned with the 'difference' the individual presented and in the majority of cases this 'difference' was

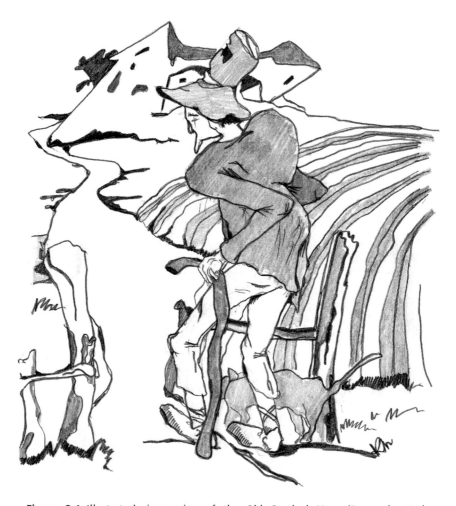

**Figure 2.1** Illustrator's impression of the Old Crooked Man. (Drawn by Kasia Halota.)

perceived as undesirable (Stiker 1999). Therefore, a concept of 'disability' was understood at some level, at least in practice, from ancient times; exclusion, marginalisation and horrific acts of violence against disabled people were prevalent.

Stiker (1999) traces ideas of sameness and difference through time; he gives a history of the idea that we ought to aspire to be the same and argues that that idea is so embedded in Western ideology today that we cannot question it. He considers, critically and in detail, the contemporary situation in light of that idea. That we ought to aspire to be alike, to conform to one particular standard, according to Stiker, is so basic a tenet of contemporary Western faith, so deeply ingrained in us, that even in our attempts to celebrate diversity, we often work to suppress it. Therefore we have identified 'disabled people' as those who are missing some necessary component of sameness, which society, through rehabilitation or prosthesis or even accommodation, must replace.

'The child is father of the man' William Wordsworth once said. Today the line is often quoted to assert that if we wish to thoroughly understand an adult, we must look at who that person was as a child.

Stiker (1999) believes that just as we look for clues to human character in earlier developmental periods, so we look for clues to societal character in earlier historical periods. Ancient Hebrew society profoundly affected the Christian tradition, ancient Greek society profoundly affected the rational tradition and both of these traditions, and others, continue to shape Western society today. Some religions supported beliefs of demonology, and the manifestation of evil spirits was the accepted explanation of disability phenomena. Certain societies in which physical prowess was viewed as necessary for defending and maintaining the community have considered a disability or deformity to be a burden, as in ancient Sparta (Wright 1980).

There are breaks in how we have historically viewed disability. In the ninth century the Mohammedans viewed disability more objectively and utilised the best scientific knowledge of the day to care for people with disabilities. Other societies such as the Greeks (Braddock and Parish 2001) have emphasised the personal worth of those with disabilities.

The older and dominant worldviews prevailed, however, and continue to shape our present view. Stiker (1999) characterised the cultural construction or dominant discourses of entire eras in European history. He believes that societies reveal themselves in the way they deal with difference. Some of the earlier worldviews will now be considered.

## Demonology

During the medieval period, some impairments were thought to have supernatural or demonological origins. Conditions such as mental illness, deafness, epilepsy and cognitive disabilities were viewed in this light. Epilepsy was associated with the devil and possession by the devil was considered the primary cause of mental illness (Braddock and Parish 2001). It was such beliefs that led to religious methods of seeking cures, exorcism being a common intervention.

People with what is now considered to be mental illness were identified as heretics by the Christian churches; many were executed and persecutions were frequently led by the Catholic Church. Persecutions included the seizure of the heretic's possessions, imprisonment, torture and execution.

During medieval times, a period thought to extend roughly from 500 AD to 1500 AD (Braddock and Parish 2001), the practice of persecuting witches (women heretics) developed gradually. Individuals with conditions that were not responsive to the conventional treatments of the time would have been regarded as witches and thousands were persecuted and executed (Braddock and Parish 2001). The term 'witch' was most commonly applied to women with mental illness.

## The Middle Ages

In the Middle Ages, physical and mental impairments were not specifically distinguished from other forms of misery or suffering. Infirmity and poverty were part of God's varied creation, the order of things. The response to difference was charity, spirituality and morality. The giving of alms, individually or through the work of institutions (hospitals, monasteries, etc.), was an exercise in virtue and suffering was a sign of divine presence. Prior to the enacting of the Poor Law in 1601, impairments of the mind or body were not specifically categorised. In fact, it is noted that deformity was not indexed, nor was it excluded, nor organised, nor especially considered: it was there and in the midst of the general miseries of 'the poor' it ought to be given mercy (Braddock and Parish 2001, Foucault 1967, Oliver 1990, Stiker 1999, Wilcock 2001).

In this system of charity, poverty and infirmity were seen as inevitable; the response was ethical rather than political or technical (although as has been previously discussed, the treatment of those with mental illness and other impairments during the early years of this period was anything but charitable). During the 4th–6th centuries monasteries and hospices for the blind were established in Turkey, Syria and France. The Belgian village of Gheel developed family care settings, offering support for people with mental illness. There were organised refuges for disabled people within existing monastic communities. Vocational opportunities in community settings were provided for the residents. Acts of charity provided an opportunity to receive blessing from God and supported the benevolent beliefs underpinning care for those with mental illness at that time. But the ethical and spiritual integration did not lead to social integration. The infirm were marginal, cared for by their families or by charitable patrons, without any social function or identity as a distinct group.

There was a relationship between poverty and disability during the Middle Ages. There was much illness generally (plague) during this time across Europe. In England records show that 75% of the population were too poor to pay taxes. Begging was commonplace and necessary. Even salaried people begged to supplement low earnings.

Disabled people begged too, but this seemed to be related to poverty rather than disability. Begging during this time was not as stigmatising as it would later become (Braddock and Parish 2001).

By the 6th century, institutions were being set up to segregate those with Hansen's disease (leprosy). Germany and Italy had hundreds of such places by the early Middle Ages.

Residential institutions were introduced to Europe by the Arabs following their conquests in Europe, particularly in Spain and France. Arabs built institutions to care for the mentally ill, believing that mental disability was divinely inspired and not demonic, as was the dominant discourse in Western society of the time. Care in their institutions was benevolent and the numbers of residents were small.

In England the Priory of St Mary's of Bethlehem was built in 1247 to provide accommodation for missionaries and visitors from abroad; it supported the physically disabled from 1330 and mentally ill from 1403. During the reign of Edward III, in 1375, the Priory was seized by the Crown and following suppression of Catholic establishments in 1539, became known as a hospital. The word 'hospital' as it is used today does not accurately convey its purpose as understood in earlier times. Such establishments were used to provide board and help to the unfortunate; these included a mix of socially and occupationally disadvantaged people of all ages as well as the poor suffering from physical or mental illness (Wilcock 2001). Today the Bethlem (as it is now known) is the longest continually operating mental hospital in Europe.

Institutions such as these were known to be very humane and wise during their early years but over time fell into disrepute and became known as places of horror. The term 'Bedlam', meaning the epitome of madness in modern speech, derives from the Bethlem. Many similar institutions during this period supplemented their upkeep by charging visitors who came to be entertained by watching the 'inmates' (Wilcock 2001).

During the Reformation many monasteries were seized by the government and as a consequence charity diminished and begging increased until the introduction of the Poor Law, outlawing begging, in 1601. Obligations were then placed on the family, local community and parishes to provide for the poor.

The Middle Ages may be summed up as holding conflicting beliefs on the origin of disability. However, as disability was so widespread at this time it was accepted as part of the natural order of things. There was a time in the West when 'fools' and others who might be called mentally ill today roamed the streets and were part of society. With the rise of rationalism and the Enlightenment, these people began to be seen as a threat and the result was the birth of institutionalisation and confinement (Wilcock 2001).

## The Age of Reason – Enlightenment

The 16th–19th centuries developed a medical as opposed to a Christian discourse on infirmity. The Enlightenment, which was the revolutionary change in thinking across Europe from the 17th century, was influenced by Francis Bacon, Isaac Newton and John Locke. Changes in thinking related to care and treatment of people with disabilities and the need to develop scientific knowledge and an ability to influence social and environmental modification. The scientific discourse had begun.

Humanism, a philosophical view and approach to life that focused on the value, dignity and potential of humans, was the dominant intellectual movement leading developments in thinking and illustrated in the arts by da Vinci, Michelangelo, Sir Thomas More and others. Advances in anatomical and physiological study fostered an interest in understanding the workings of the body and a mechanistic and reductionist discourse began to develop (Braddock and Parish 2001, Wilcock 2001). During this period there was a change from seeking supernatural causes of disability to seeking a scientific explanation or reason, although belief in supernatural causes of mental illness continued to persist throughout the 16th century and ended officially with the repeal of the Witchcraft Acts in 1736.

Begging was outlawed and so disabled people lost an important means of income. Additionally, the status which beggars previously had, that of a means by which almsgivers could please God, was gone. The outlawing of begging marginalised the disabled, who were no longer as visible in the community. Ideas about poverty began to change and impairments began to be seen as not just the natural order of things but a curse. In the 18th century, madhouses and criminal prisons were combined facilities and increased numbers of the mentally ill were being committed (Braddock and Parish 2001, Wilcock 2001).

By the 18th century the concern was less to explain than to describe and make an inventory of impairments. The 17th century saw the beginning of confinement in hospitals. Whereas earlier, disabled people had been aggregated with the poor (not only as objects of charity in the Middle Ages, but under the Poor Laws of the 16th century in England), now institutions specifically for disabled people were established. Families cared for those with motor and intellectual difficulties, and only if they were unable to do so were people handed over to institutions for the poor, the old and the infirm. Confinement within institutions was never so general for people with sensory and motor impairments as it was for the mentally ill.

There was a concern with classification of disorders, disabilities and infirmities. In many cases this classification seemed to be for the benefit of legal practices rather than for treatment purposes. The philosopher Francis Bacon noted in 1605 that the superstition of the Middle Ages and

Renaissance contributed nothing to knowledge. Bacon introduced the notion of scientific and systematic study and experimentation. His approach was to dominate psychological research for the next 300 years. It was also during this time that the professional classes began their ascendancy, key amongst them being medicine and education. Disability became medicalised and professionalised and became the interest of others during this time. Following a parliamentary inquiry it was discovered that there were glaring deficiencies between practice and what was recommended in theory (Braddock and Parish 2001, Wilcock 2001).

The idea of education or re-education of disabled people was a product of 18th-century Enlightenment thinking. It was during this time that a general European interest developed in the capacities of the impaired. Sign language for deaf people was introduced as was education for blind people (Louis Braille was a student at the first French establishment). The 18th century also saw the proliferation of residential schools for deaf and blind people. Manualism and oralism developed as the primary means of educating the deaf and the conflicts between these opposing systems became increasingly energetic. The polemic continues to pose difficulty despite signed communication being the preference of the majority of deaf people. The education offered was comprehensive, with the best examples being provided in France and Spain. The first school for deaf people in the United States, the American Asylum for the Education of the Deaf and Dumb, was opened in 1817 by Thomas Gallaudet and Laurent Clerc. The well-known Gallaudet University is part of this legacy (Braddock and Parish 2001, Wilcock 2001).

## Moral treatment

By the 19th century there were educational establishments for the deaf and the blind, and orthopaedic institutions were established with techniques and machines for correcting the body. During a period from 1792 to around the late 1800s care of the mentally ill became more humane; meaningful occupation began to be prescribed for patients and an association between occupation and health began to emerge. The prime mover in this ideological shift was William Tuke (1732–1822) and later his grandson Samuel Tuke (1784–1857) continued to develop his ideas. In 1792 Tuke opened the Retreat in York, a facility for the mentally ill which advocated the provision of meaningful occupation as a therapeutic intervention, rather than forced labour. This period is recognised as the birth of the occupational therapy profession (Wilcock 2001). Later these ideals were developed in France and the United States. Moral treatment was acclaimed on both sides of the Atlantic and for a brief period, care of the mentally ill was humane in focus.

However, due to overcrowding in asylums the therapeutic aspect of the regime began to decline and the moral treatment approach began to disappear (Braddock and Parish 2001, Wilcock 2001). Overcrowding of criminals into the psychiatric asylums led to their downfall and many gaols wanted to release their prisoners to the new facilities built for the mentally ill. In later decades, moral treatment gave way to custodial care and a belief that mental illness could not be cured. Asylums grew in size and number and were often the agents of severe abuse to inmates (Braddock and Parish 2001, Wilcock 2001).

## Freak shows

The onset of the Industrial Revolution saw a change in the pattern of work within community life. A move towards mechanisation and away from the earlier feudal systems of work and a decline in the 'cottage' industries common prior to this time had profound implications for the disabled of a community. The change from small family/community-based enterprises to the factory and institutional work settings made care/support of the vulnerable within a community difficult, if not impossible, in many cases. Migration and fragmentation of extended families in search of work, resulting from the changing work patterns heralded by the Industrial Revolution, raised questions concerning the practical care of the vulnerable in a community – a group which hitherto had uniquely defined roles within the smaller family enterprises.

'Human oddities' were exhibited in museums, circuses, fairs, freak shops and shows in 19th-century Europe and America. 'Freaks', the term used at the time, included people billed as primitive and exotic, as well as those with physical and mental abnormalities: bearded ladies, 'pinheads' (microcephalics), Siamese twins, 'half men' (people missing limbs), dwarfs and giants.

Today freak shows seem anachronistic, an indecent exploitation of those with disabilities. But one 'freak' has made it to our time with particular force: Joseph Merrick, the Elephant man, discovered in a freak show by a London doctor in 1884. Merrick suffered from a rare disease that progressively deformed his facial structure and body, inhibiting his movements and rendering him so grotesque that normal social intercourse was impossible. Joseph Merrick had been transformed from a suffering individual to an exhibit, a shape-shifting curiosity whose different guises suited his intended audiences. Even the doctor Frederick Treves, who brings us closer to Merrick than anyone else, consistently refers to Merrick by the wrong name – John instead of Joseph. Treves presents Merrick as a victim whose personhood was denied in being exhibited as a freak (Ingstad and Reynolds-White 1995). Yet with the changes in social organisation and family groupings consequent upon the Industrial Revolution, the 'freak shows' provided one way in which disabled groups, hitherto supported by family networks, could make a living, however unethical this may seem today. Freak shows were popular throughout the 19th century, as they reinforced the normality of the viewer, and continued in parts of the United States until the 1940s (Braddock and Parish 2001, Wilcock 2001).

## The 20th century

World War I marked the beginning of rehabilitation as we know it. As prostheses were developed, so also arose the general notions of replacement, substitution and compensation which in time were applied to all congenital and acquired impairments. The process was not one of curing but of replacement. It is during this period that we see the denial of difference, whereas earlier epochs situated the infirm as exceptional in some way (Braddock and Parish 2001).

Segregation became common in Europe by the mid-19th century and schools continued to develop, particularly those for physically disabled children in which the focus was primarily on industrial training. Louis Braille developed a standard dot code communication for blind people and an intimate link between the fields of deafness was understood. Different educational styles began to emerge such as Montessori, sensory-motor training, intellectual training and moral training and socialisation (Braddock and Parish 2001).

The British Deaf Association (BDA) was the first political action group formed to promote the needs and rights of the Deaf community. This group had great pride and a strong sense of identity.

Exploitation and the availability of resident labour in mental hospitals meant that many were able to become self-managing and self-funding. Abuse of inmates was commonplace in many institutions of the time and included such interventions as sterilisation, as support for the eugenics movement and social Darwinism grew. Some mentally ill people became targets for medical experiments; in one such experiment food containing radioactive elements was given to patients in a mental institution in Massachusetts as recently as the 1950s (Braddock and Parish 2001).

The concept that cure was not possible and that life-long custodial care was necessary became the routine intervention and the removal of those with mental illness from society contributed to the consolidation of segregation. Institutions that could house in excess of 2000 inmates were built. Social control and repression of disabled people was the dominant discourse during this time.

Physical disabilities were commonplace, often due to industrial injury or military service, and compensation became payable although those with mental illness were not eligible. Service men returning from World War I were eligible for rehabilitation programmes in a bid to get back to employment.

In the field of intellectual disabilities some progress was made in the USA despite the Depression and World War II. Foster family care was introduced in the 1930s and research has shown many beneficial effects from this (Braddock and Parish 2001). Community-based mental health programmes began to develop in the 1940s following bad reports from the mental hospitals and influenced by the film 'The Snake Pit'. Mental health legislation was enacted to protect patients (Barnes, 1992, Braddock and Parish 2001, Wilcock 2001).

In summary, a brief historical perspective of disability and the influence of capitalism as outlined by Finkelstein (Oliver 1990) in his 'historical materialist model' suggests three phases of historical development.

- Phase I – Britain before the Industrial Revolution: feudal society.
- Phase II – industrialisation when the focus of work shifted from home to factory: capitalist society. Morris (Oliver 1990) states that changes in the organisation of work, from a rural-based, co-operative system where individuals contributed what they could to the production process to an urban, factory-based one organised around the individual waged labourer, had profound consequences. The operation of the labour market in the 19th century effectively depressed disabled people of all kinds to the bottom of the market.
- Phase III – the transition to socialism (yet to be realised) which will see the liberation of disabled people from the segregative practices of society largely as a result of new technologies and the working together of professionals and disabled people towards common goals.

## Anthropological perspectives

The term 'discourses' as used by anthropologists is a way of objectifying situations, issues, values, people and relationships. In the common use of the term, discourses 'say' something and institutional practices imply something; at some level a message is conveyed.

Frazer's (1971) anthropological work *The Golden Bough* presents many examples of negative treatment, oppression and flagrant abuse of people with disabilities. In some parts of the East Indian islands it is thought that epilepsy can be cured by striking the patient on the face with the leaves of certain trees and then throwing them away, thus ridding themselves of the evil. There is a worldwide superstition that by injuring footprints, you injure the feet that made them. Thus natives of south-eastern Australia think they can lame a man by placing sharp pieces of quartz, glass, bone or charcoal in his footprints. Rheumatic pains are often attributed to this cause.

Anthropological research in the field of disability has been slow. Much research in medical anthropology has a therapeutic theme. It has concentrated on perceptions of illness and disease, on modes of healing, and on the interaction between patient and practitioner. Studies of disability require us to move away from the clinic toward the community, where individuals with families live with deficits. We are less concerned with disease than with its long-term consequences and more concerned with adjustment than with therapy.

Ingstad and Reynolds-White (1995) note that impairment raises moral and metaphysical problems about personhood, responsibility and the meaning of differences. Questions about autonomy and dependence, capacity and identity, and the meaning of loss are central. One of the basic questions for cross-cultural research on disability is that of how biological impairments relate to personhood and to culturally defined differences among persons.

Studies have described (Ingstad and Reynolds-White 1995) the invalidation and infantilisation of disabled people; one's validity as a full person is denied. Being 'different' means being less. In Western culture today the term 'invalid' is applied to many disabled people, clearly a perceived view of their worth in society. A distinction is made between humanity and personhood.

Despite the fact that accessibility is a positive aspect for a large part of the population, it is still looked upon as a field of specialised care. Commentators have drawn attention to the use of the word 'they' when referring to disabled people (Barton and Oliver 1997, Berger and Luckmann 1996, Braddock and Parish 2001, Rioux 1997, Somers 1994). The use of the personal pronoun 'they' marks and strengthens the dissociation of disabled persons, and this dissociation indicates that people with disabilities are exposed to an alienating process of being categorised. Through this process disabled people are marked as a group different from others, consisting of similar human beings without individual features. This dissociated group is then being characterised by particular properties, something which is common when we speak of *the others* – irrespective of whom this category consists of. These both conscious and unconscious psychological processes, it is proposed, suggest a social contempt of weakness, believed to be deeply rooted in our Western culture.

Our conscious and more unconscious reflections in this area are mirrored by the use of the words 'elderly and disabled'. Elderly people who are dependent on a walking frame will sometimes dispute the fact that they are disabled. Young disabled persons also reject being mentioned together with elderly people. There are good reasons for these protests, because young and old are often put into the same service system. However, our general tendency not to accept getting old also exists as an idea among people with disabilities.

In the paradigm of 'planning for our future selves', there is, in many ways, a new comprehension that the consideration of disabled people in planning does not only imply *the others*, but is actually a more realistic understanding of the entirety of our lives (Center for Universal Design 1997).This signifies a comprehension rather than a displacement of the fact that we are all getting old and thereby more disabled.

The cultural conceptualisation of humanity is variable; the anomalies that may be seen as inhuman differ greatly from one society to another, and they do not correspond directly to Western biomedical definitions of impairment. Twins are not considered human by the Punan Bah of Central Borneo nor are children born with teeth by the Bariba of East Africa. Accounts from some societies suggest that individuals with certain kinds of impairments or biological characteristics may not be considered human. Or rather, there may be a point at which such an individual's humanity may be in doubt. In many northern countries (i.e. Western), the abortion of a defective fetus is considered more acceptable than that of a 'normal' one, suggesting that the human status of an impaired individual is more negotiable. The debate about whether severely impaired infants or even adults should be kept alive involves the attribution of humanity.

If 'personhood' is seen as being not simply human but human in a way that is valued and meaningful then individuals can be seen as persons to a greater or lesser extent. There is a growing consciousness in Europe and North America of disablement as a human and social issue that touches us all, the disabled and 'temporarily abled' as well.

Impairments of the mind, the senses and the motor functioning of the body are universal. Everywhere there are people who live with biological defects that cannot be cured and that inhibit, to some extent, their ability to perform certain functions. But the significance of a deficit always depends on more than its biological nature; it is shaped by the human circumstances in which it exists (Ingstad and Reynolds-Whyte 1995).

# References

Barnes C (1992) *Disabling Imagery and The Media*. Ryburn, Halifax.

Barton M, Oliver M (1997) *Disability Studies: past, present and future*. Disability Press, Leeds.

Berger PL, Luckmann T (1996) *The Social Construction of Reality*. Doubleday, New York.

Braddock D, Parish S (2001) An institutional history of disability. In: Albrecht GL, Seelman KD, Bury M (eds) (2001) *Handbook Of Disability Studies*. Sage Publications, California.

Center for Universal Design (1997) *The Principles of Universal Design* (Version 2.0). North Carolina State University, Raleigh, North Carolina.

Cone AA (1998) Self-advocacy in the United States: historical overview and future vision. In: Wehman P, Kregel J (eds) *More Than a Job: securing satisfying careers for people with disabilities*. Paul H. Brookes Publishing, Baltimore, Maryland.

Foucault M (1969) What is an author? In: Rabinow P (ed) *The Foucault Reader*. Penguin, Harmondsworth, Middlesex.

Frazer JG (1971) *The Golden Bough: a study in magic and religion*. Macmillan, Basingstoke.

Gergen KJ (1999) *An Invitation to Social Construction*. Sage, Thousand Oaks, California.

Greene GJ, Lee MY (2002) The social construction of empowerment. In: O'Melia M, Miley KK (eds) *Pathways to Power: readings in contextual social work practice*. Allyn and Bacon, Boston, Massachusetts, pp.175–201.

Heron J, Reason P (1997) A participatory inquiry paradigm. *Qualitative Inquiry* **3(3)**, 274–295.

Ingstad B, Reynolds-Whyte S (1995) *Disability and Culture*. University of California Press, Berkeley, California.

Kroll (1973) A reappraisal of psychiatry in the Middle Ages. *Archives of General Psychiatry* **29**, 276–283.

Laird J (1993) *Revisioning Social Work Education: a social constructionist approach*. Haworth Press, New York.

Mills S (2005) Discourse. *Literary Encyclopedia*. Literary Dictionary Company. Available at: www.litencic.com/php/stopics.php?rec=true&UID=1261.

Oliver M (1990) *The Politics of Disablement: critical texts in social work and the welfare state*. Macmillan Press, London.

Rioux M (1997) When myths masquerade as science: disability research from an equality-rights perspective. In: Barton L, Oliver M (eds) *Disability Studies: past, present and future*. Disability Press, Leeds.

Somers M (1994) The narrative construction of identity: a relational and network approach. *Theory and Society* **23**, 605–649.

Stiker HJ (1999) *A History of Disability* (trans. Sayers W). University of Michigan Press, Ann Arbor, Michigan.

Wilcock A (2001) *Occupation for Health Volume 1: a journey from self health to prescription*. Lavenham Press, Suffolk.

Wright GN (1980) *Total Rehabilitation*. Little, Brown, Boston, Massachusetts.

# 3: Theories and models of disability

In the previous chapter the nature of knowledge and understanding relating to disability was presented. The influence of folklore on primitive communities' perceptions of disability and the shift in disability discourse from medieval times through the Enlightenment and into modern times have combined to underpin our contemporary understanding of disability and mould our expectations of the role of disabled people within our communities. The process is an iterative one, comprising imperceptible changes over time, and although the perception and status of disabled people have changed and evolved, equal status with the able-bodied is elusive and has yet to be achieved. Disabled people have been dehumanised and marginalised within the characters of folklore, feared as supernatural beings or with supernatural associations, they have been pitied and despised in medieval times, studied and classified in the Age of Enlightenment and segregated and excluded in modern times.

In order to better understand the complexities underpinning our present perceptions of disability and the means by which our institutional, social and charitable organisations orientate themselves towards disabled people, an exploration of the theories and models that underpin the construct will be presented in this chapter.

## The function of theories and models

### Theories

Francis Bacon (1561–1626) claimed that theories arise as a result of inductive knowledge (i.e. the collection of facts and experimentation) and the acceptance as true of the stated generalisations to explain relationships. If unchallenged, these relationships attain the status of laws and principles.

Karl Popper, a philosopher of science, suggested in his book *The Logic of Scientific Discovery* (1959) that a theory is no more than a conjecture or hypothesis, but it generates deductions which can be tested. Theories therefore can be disproven when future tests show them to be false. He presents an opposing view to Bacon's, suggesting that since a challenge may always be mounted to inductive knowledge (it takes but one observation or experiment to discount a generalisation) such arguments will always be fallacious. The best theories are those that have high information content, thus making them testable and therefore potentially falsifiable (Young and Quinn 1992). Theories therefore cannot be accepted as fact or true, they merely provide human explanations for events and are thus subject to logical analysis, yet they are the most powerful tools we have for understanding the world. Our understanding of the construct of disability is likewise grounded in theory which as we have seen is fallacious. Those theories whose predictions are easily testable tend to be predominantly reductionist (Young and Quinn 1992).

Popper further postulates that if social theories are to be credible they must contain hypotheses whose predictions can be tested. He proposes that all our theories, philosophical and personal, should be subjected to criticism so that they lose their dogmatic quality and become more objective and representative of the truth. Such opinion holds a particular challenge for practitioners in the fields of health, education, social care, design and others; we are urged to adopt a critical attitude to the dogma or orthodoxy in our fields of endeavour. Popper is critical of the professional who hesitates to challenge dogma and who accepts a theory unquestioningly in keeping with the prevailing 'zeitgeist' for their time (Young and Quinn 1992).

The position we hold in relation to perspectives on disability is subject to the processes outlined above. Knowledge generation and the organisation of the world consequent to that understanding and belief are complex, resulting from many formulations and reformulations of hypotheses and providing us with a strong conceptualisation of the present-day construct of disability. The place disability occupies in a world so constructed clearly derives from the prevailing theories in a given time and place. Theories, as we have seen, are fallible.

Almost all studies of disability have a grand theory underpinning them (Oliver 1990). That grand theory can be characterised as 'the personal tragedy theory'. The social world differs from the natural world in at least one fundamental respect: human beings give meanings to objects in the social world and subsequently orientate their behaviour towards these objects in terms of the meanings given to them. In other words, as far as disability is concerned, if it is seen as a tragedy, then disabled people will be treated as if they are the victims of some tragic happening or occurrence. This treatment will occur not just in everyday interactions but will be translated into social policies which will attempt to compensate these victims for the tragedies that have befallen them. It has fallen to disabled people themselves both to provide critiques of this implicit theory and to construct their own alternatives, which might be called 'social oppression theory' (Oliver 1990, Swain *et al.* 2003).

Alternatively, it logically follows that if disability is defined as social oppression, then disabled people will be seen as the collective victims of an uncaring society rather than as individual victims of circumstance. Such a view will be translated into social policies geared towards alleviating oppression rather than compensating individuals. At present the individual and tragic view of disability dominates both social interactions and social policies.

## Models

Models may be described as a means of representing an aspect of the natural world in some familiar way so that our understanding of the complex element can be improved. In this text we will explore the nature and utility of models as an aid to our understanding of knowledge from a particular stance.

There are many different types of models, physical, symbolic and iconic, many of which are common across a range of settings and disciplines. The toys of childhood were the first encounter with models for most of us. Physical models include those of the health educator; anatomical models representing bodily organs and structure are familiar to students and help to provide a better understanding of the body's form and function. There are also the iconic models of the geographer; globes, maps and atlases represent an abstraction of the world or of an aspect of it. The designer and architect improve their understanding of a building or artefact through the use of plans and designs. The scientist's and mathematician's understanding of their realm is enhanced through the use of symbolic models such as graphs and formulas. Academic disciplines also use theoretical and conceptual models to strengthen understanding of particular knowledge (Young and Quinn 1992).

In the evolution of our understanding of disability many models have been applied. Some of those influencing the construct today will be critically considered in this chapter. Practitioners and professionals should develop a lively awareness of how these overarching models of disability influence their practice and the interpretation of their profession's professional models. Professional practice models will be explored in greater detail in Chapter 4.

### Applications and interpretations

Models of disability are tools for defining impairment and, ultimately, for providing a basis upon which government and society can devise strategies for meeting the needs of disabled people (Morris 1991, Oliver 1990). They are often treated with scepticism as it is thought that they do not reflect the real world, are often incomplete and encourage narrow thinking, and seldom offer detailed guidance for action. However, they are a useful framework in which to gain an understanding of disability issues, and also of the perspective held by those creating and applying the models (Morris 1991, Oliver 1990, Swain *et al.* 2003).

Models of disability are essentially devised by people about other people. They provide an insight into the attitudes, conceptions and beliefs of the former and how they impact on the latter. Models reveal the ways in which our society provides or limits access to work, goods, services, economic influence and political power for people with disabilities (Morris 1991, Oliver 1990, Swain *et al.* 2003).

Models are influenced by two fundamental philosophies. The first sees disabled people as dependent upon society. This can result in paternalism, segregation and discrimination. The second perceives disabled people as customers of what society has to offer. This leads to choice, empowerment, equality of human rights and integration. As we examine the different models, we will see the degree to which each philosophy has been applied (Oliver 1990).

## The medical model

The medical model holds that disability results from an individual person's physical or mental limitations, and is largely unconnected to social or geographical environments. It is sometimes referred to as the biological inferiority or functional limitation model. It is illustrated by the World Health Organization's (WHO) definitions, which were devised by doctors as follows (WHO 1980).

- *Impairment*: any loss or abnormality of psychological or anatomical structure or function.
- *Disability*: any restriction or lack of ability (resulting from an impairment) to perform an activity in the manner or within the range considered normal for a human being.
- *Handicap*: any disadvantage for a given individual, resulting from impairment or a disability that limits or prevents the fulfilment of a role that is normal for that individual.

From this, it is easy to see how people with disabilities might become stigmatised as 'lacking' or 'abnormal' (WHO 2002).

The medical model places the source of the problem within a single impaired person and concludes that solutions are found by focusing on the individual. A more sophisticated form of the model allows for economic factors and recognises that a poor economic climate will adversely affect a disabled person's work opportunities (Altman 2001). Even so, it still seeks a solution within the individual by helping him or her overcome personal impairment to cope with a faltering labour market. In simplest terms, the medical model assumes that the first step solution is to find a cure or, to use WHO terminology, make disabled people more 'normal'. This invariably fails because disabled people are not necessarily sick or cannot be improved by remedial treatment. The only remaining solution is to accept the 'abnormality' and provide the necessary care to support the 'incurable' impaired person. Policy makers are limited to a range of options based upon a programme of rehabilitation, vocational training for employment, income maintenance programmes and the provision of aids and equipment.

This functional limitation, also known as the Nagi (medical), model has dominated the formulation of disability policy for years. Although we should not reject out of hand its therapeutic aspects which may cure or alleviate the physical and mental condition of many disabled people, it does not offer a realistic perspective from the viewpoint of disabled people themselves (Bickenbach 2001). To begin with, most would reject the concept of being 'abnormal'. Also, the model imposes a paternalistic approach to problem solving which, although well intentioned, concentrates on 'care' and ultimately provides justification for institutionalisation and segregation. This restricts disabled people's opportunities to make choices, control their lives and develop their potential (Morris 2003).

Finally, the model fosters existing prejudices in the minds of employers. Because the condition is 'medical', a disabled person will *ipso facto* be prone to ill health and sick leave, is likely to deteriorate and will be less productive than work colleagues.

The WHO revised its definition of disability in 2002 within the *International Classification of Functioning, Disability and Health*, more commonly known as ICF. This definition, developed by the stakeholders, including not only health and social care professionals but also service users and carers, interprets disability more broadly; its focus is on health, functioning and participation. The ICF will be explored more fully in Chapter 9.

## The expert/professional model

The expert/professional model has provided a traditional response to disability issues and can be seen as an offshoot of the medical model.

Within its framework, professionals follow a process of identifying the impairment and its limitations (using the medical model) and taking the necessary action to improve the position of the disabled person. This has tended to produce a system in which an authoritarian, overactive service provider prescribes and acts for a passive client (Conway 2000).

This relationship has been described as that of fixer (the professional) and fixee (the client), and clearly contains an inequality that limits collaboration. Although a professional may be caring, the imposition of solutions can be less than benevolent. If the decisions are made by the 'expert', the client has no choice and is unable to exercise the basic human right of freedom in his or her own actions. At the extreme, it undermines the client's dignity by removing the ability to participate in the simplest, everyday decisions affecting his or her life (Oliver 1990, Swain *et al.* 2003).

## The health psychology model

This model, also known as the self-regulation model, developed within a paramedical perspective on disability, recognises the psychosocial components of health. It acknowledges that disability cannot simply be reduced to impairment because the extent and degree of disability cannot be directly predicted from impairment alone. This model views disability within the context of the value a disabled person attributes to the lost functions associated with the impairment and how the disabled person copes with the lost function (Bickenbach 2001). For instance, if a disabled person is unable to get out of bed then this implies that they will be unable to get to the shops; if a disabled person is unable to use the toilet independently, this lost function may be rated more highly than that expected from the impairment alone. This model focuses on coping with and adjusting to the 'trauma' and 'loss' associated with the impairment and on developing strategies to minimise its disabling effects. The focus of intervention is on encouraging the disabled person to understand and manage their emotional response to disability. It does not directly address the disability itself or offer an explanation of disability (Swain *et al.* 2003).

## The self-regulation model

The self-regulation model is mediated by two factors. The first is mental representations of impairment, e.g. cause, cure, consequences, suggesting that the disabled person will develop the appropriate coping behaviour. Coping behaviour according to this model generally means following expectations, e.g. adhering to a rehabilitation programme.

However, representations do not reliably predict coping behaviour and so this model has been extended to encompass a second variable; the factors that govern behavioural intention are explicitly identified. These are attitude to behaviour, subjective norm for behaviour and perceived control over behaviour. This gives a more powerful explanation of the impairment–disability relationship (Bickenbach 2001, Swain *et al.* 2003).

The problems with this model are that there is often a lack of relationship between intention and actual behaviour; also the model fails to consider the impact of the environment, both social and physical, as a potential source of psychological problems. Although the model goes beyond the deterministic impairment–disability causation, the problem is viewed as remaining firmly rooted within the individual. The duty is placed on the individual to adapt to their circumstances with no expectation for change placed upon society or the environment (Swain *et al.* 2003).

## The social cognition model

We interpret the social world in the same way we do the world of objects; the principles of the information processing model still apply (Grieve 2000). The brain can be represented as a limited capacity system which has the task of making sense of unlimited, unstructured, sensory data and to do this efficiently the brain divides the world into categories for 'cognitive economy'. People use a number of common strategies to make sense of the world, as a means to organise 'messy' social information without having to process data exhaustively. These strategies work well in most situations but inherent in this process is the tendency for the development of bias and stereotypes.

Stereotypes are thought to be a product of the natural categorisation processes involved in perception and cognition – a negative or positive stereotype develops from a category consisting mainly of negative or positive attributes. Since the dominant view of disabled people is that of 'personal tragedy', a negative stereotype of disabled people emerges. Associated with categorical differentiation is the phenomenon of 'spread' which may be described as the process whereby when a person is assigned to a particular category, they become linked to other negative attributes of the category even when there is no connection to the disabled person (Albrecht *et al.* 2001, Morris 2003). Spread accounts for the tendency to speak louder to a blind person or to talk 'down' to a person with quadriplegia, because we link them to a more general category of disability.

Impairment is often more salient to able-bodied than it is to disabled people. It is often assumed that a disabled person can never feel part of the 'normal' community due to assumptions that disability dominates his or her life. But this view of the disabled casts them in the role of the sad, pathetic, angry, bitter, heroic and tragic player in society's drama. We have seen how disabled people are categorised, set apart according to their impairment due to the pervasiveness of the medical model definitions. Such categorisations lead to prejudice against those considered as being outside the 'in group'. Social categorisation leads to the formation of positive categories as defined against various other groups (out groups). Our self-image and how we are viewed by others will therefore be determined by how we view ourselves and how we are viewed by others in relation to these groups (Swain *et al.* 2003).

There is evidence that our unfavourable impressions of disabled people (or indeed any minority and/or stigmatised group) become less when we develop greater familiarity with that group through providing opportunity for contact. This is known as the contact hypothesis (Allport 1954).

One problem with social cognition is that since the information processing (Grieve 2000) takes place within the brain of an individual, it cannot be considered to be 'social' or a social process. As the disabled person takes the role of the information being processed they continue to occupy the focus of the gaze of others. The contact hypothesis predicts change in the attitudes of an individual who comes into prolonged contact with a member of a stigmatised group, although the hypothesis does not explain how this would impact in any broader cultural context. The model fails to address the emotional factors involved in prejudice, such as the fear of the able-bodied of becoming disabled themselves (Morris 2003).

## The tragedy/charity model

The rise of traditional voluntary organisations can be linked to the rise of capitalism itself and by the middle of the 19th century there were a considerable number of small societies for the blind in existence (Braddock and Parish 2001). Throughout the latter half of the century similar organisations grew up for the welfare of the 'deaf' and 'crippled'. The growth in these organisations signified a move away from 'individual concern for the handicapped' to a concern for the welfare of particular groups, and such groups were successful in raising public awareness and encouraging the state to take on particular responsibilities. These groups were effective and even after the establishment of the welfare state, the state was happy to allow voluntary organisations to continue to provide services, sometimes in partnership and sometimes as sole providers.

Over time it became apparent that disabled people were not having all of their needs met. As most of these organisations are registered charities, direct and overt political activity is precluded (Braddock and Parish 2001, Oliver and Barnes 2003). These organisations have built up a relationship with the establishment which gives them credibility but little power. This credibility has been based upon history and tradition rather than representativness of these organisations, whose 'key decision makers' are usually salaried professional staff who articulate their own assumptions about the needs of disabled people rather than the needs of disabled people as they themselves see them.

Disillusionment spread amongst disabled people and several single-issue pressure groups formed which led to the emergence of the disability movement. The disability movement has been the prime mover in the development of the social model of disability (Oliver 1990).

The tragedy/charity model depicts disabled people as victims of circumstance, deserving of pity. This and the medical model are probably those most used by non-disabled people to define and explain disability (Swain *et al.* 2003). The tragedy/charity model is condemned by its critics as dis-enabling and the cause of much discrimination. Over 400,000 adults in Great Britain are affected by institutionalisation. Given the choice, many, if not most, would opt for community life with adequate support.

Employers will view disabled people as charitable cases. Rather than address the real issues of creating a workplace conducive to the employment of people with disabilities, employers may conclude that making charitable donations meets social and economic obligations (Oliver 1990).

## The economic model

Under this model, disability is defined by the perception of a person's inability to participate in work. It also assesses the degree to which impairment affects an individual's productivity and the economic consequences for the individual, employer and state. Such consequences include loss of earnings for and payment for assistance by the individual, lower profit margins for the employer, and state welfare payments (Morris 1991, 2003, Oliver 1990).

The economic model is used primarily by policy makers to assess distribution of benefits to those who are unable to participate fully in work. In recent years, however, the preoccupation with productivity has conflicted with the application of the medical model to classify disability to counter fraudulent benefit claims, leading to confusion and a lack of co-ordination in disablement policy.

The two key difficulties with this model are firstly, the stigma that the disabled person experiences by the underlining of their inability to match the performance of work colleagues, and secondly the difficulties in accurately assessing the correct level of subsidy to give employers (Swain *et al.* 2003).

The emergence of social enterprise initiatives and, in particular, social firms across Europe and the UK may provide one solution to this difficulty (Reynolds and McDermid 2007, Warner 2006). It is beyond the scope of this text to discuss social firms in any great detail but an overview is offered. The reader is encouraged to refer to the original sources for a more in-depth and critical account of these initiatives.

The social firm model developed in Italy in the 1970s for people with psychiatric disabilities. It spread widely throughout Italy and continues to thrive there. The model later gained prominence throughout Europe. Known as 'affirmative businesses' in North America, social firms are businesses created to employ people with a broad range of disabilities or those who are disadvantaged in the labour market in some way.

The underlying principles of social firms are:

■ up to one-third of employees are from disabled or otherwise disadvantaged groups
■ all employees receive a market wage not less than the national hourly minimum rate
■ the business operates without subsidy.

Social firms have developed across Europe including the UK, Ireland, Germany, Sweden, Netherlands, Spain and Greece and internationally have grown in Canada, Australia, Japan and North America although growth has been slower in the US than elsewhere. One reason for this may be the growth of the successful alternative supported employment model and/or the different social security provision in the US compared to the other countries listed (Warner 2006). The most successful firms are those that are able to identify a market niche, produce/provide labour-intensive products that have a public orientation for the business and have links to treatment services (Warner 2006). Some social firms have been awarded government and other national contracts. Such initiatives help social firms to grow although not all countries adopt these favourable practices (Reynolds and McDermid 2007).

The Council of Europe Action Plan 2006–2015 recommends the development of more social firms/enterprises throughout Europe (Council of Europe 2006). It is likely therefore that in the not too distant future this sector is set to grow.

## The customer/empowering model

This is the opposite of the expert model. Here, the professional is viewed as a service provider to the disabled client and his or her family. The client selects what services they believe are appropriate whilst the service provider acts as consultant, coach and resource provider (Conway 2000, Swain *et al.* 2003).

Recent operations of this model have placed financial resources in the control of the client, who may choose to purchase state or private care or both (Oliver 1990). One manifestation of this model in action is the growing number of direct payment schemes and use of Advance Directives around the UK (Swain *et al.* 2003).

## The religious model

The religious model views disability as a punishment inflicted upon an individual or family by an external force (Braddock and Parish 2001). It can be due to misdemeanours committed by the disabled person, someone in the family or community group, or forebears. Birth conditions can be due to actions committed in a previous reincarnation (Schoon-Eberly 1988).

Sometimes the presence of 'evil spirits' is used to explain differences in behaviour, especially in conditions such as schizophrenia. Acts of exorcism or sacrifice may be performed to expel or placate the negative influence, or recourse made to persecution or even death of the individual who is 'different'.

In some cases, the disability stigmatises a whole family, lowering their status or even leading to total social exclusion. Or it can be interpreted as an individual's inability to conform within a family structure. Conversely, it can be seen as a necessary affliction to be suffered before some future spiritual reward (Schoon-Eberly 1988).

## The social model

The social model of disability proposes the following as definitions of disability from both the medical model and social model perspectives.

### Medical model

▪ *Disability:* physical or mental impairment which has a substantial and long-term adverse effect on a person's ability to carry out normal day-to-day activities.

## Social model

- *Impairment:* lacking part or all of a limb, or having a defective limb, organism or mechanism of the body.
- *Disability:* the disadvantage or restriction of activity caused by a contemporary social organisation which takes little or no account of people who have physical impairments and thus excludes them from the mainstream of social activities (Finkelstein 1976).
- *Handicap:* the United Nations 'World Program of Action Concerning Disabled Persons' defines handicap as 'a function of the relationship between disabled persons and their environments. It occurs when they encounter cultural, physical or social barriers which prevent their access to the various systems of society that are available to other citizens' (Ratzka 2002).

The social model views disability as a consequence of environmental, social and attitudinal barriers that prevent people with impairments from maximum participation in society. Its philosophy originates in the US civil rights movement and it has been championed by the British Council of Organisations of Disabled People and Rights Now, which calls for self-determination. It is advocated in the UK by leading thinkers such as Dr Steven Duckworth and Bert Massie and has been the guiding light for the the Local Government Management Board and the establishment of the new Commission for Disabled People (Oliver and Barnes 2003).

It is also referred to as the minority-group model of disability. This argues from a sociopolitical viewpoint that disability stems from the failure of society to adjust to meet the needs and aspirations of a disabled minority. This presents a radically different perspective on disability issues and parallels the doctrine of those concerned with racial equality that 'racism is a problem of whites from which blacks suffer'. If the problem lies with society and the environment, then society and environment must change. If a wheelchair user cannot use a bus, the bus must be redesigned.

To support the argument, short-sighted people living in the UK are not classified as disabled. Eye tests and visual aids – which are either affordable or freely available – mean that this impairment does not prevent them participating fully in the life of the community. If, however, they live in a third-world country where such eye care is not available they are severely disabled. The inability to read and subsequently learn and gather information would be counted as a severe impairment in any society.

This model implies that the removal of attitudinal, physical and institutional barriers will improve the lives of disabled people, giving them the same opportunities as others on an equitable basis. Taken to its logical conclusion, there would be no disability within a fully developed society.

The strength of this model lies in its placing the onus upon society and not the individual. At the same time it focuses on the needs of the individual whereas the medical model uses diagnoses to produce categories of disability and assumes that people with the same impairment have identical needs and abilities. It also offers positive solutions that have been proved to work in, for example, Canada, Australia and the USA (Seelman 2001).

The model faces two challenges. Firstly, as the population gets older the numbers of people with impairments will rise, making it harder for society to adjust. Secondly, its concepts can be difficult to understand, particularly by dedicated professionals in the fields of charities and rehabilitation. These have to be persuaded that their role must change from that of 'cure or care' to a less obtrusive one of helping disabled people to take control of their own lives (Barnes and Mercer 2001).

The social model's limitations arise from its failure to emphasise certain aspects of disability. Morris (1991) adds a further dimension: 'While environmental barriers and social attitudes are a crucial part of our experience of disability – and do indeed disable us – to suggest that this is all there is, is to deny the personal experience of physical and intellectual restrictions, of illness or the fear of dying'. Black disabled people face problems of both racial and disability discrimination within a system of service provision designed by white able-bodied people for white disabled people (Bickenbach 2001).

## The social adapted model

This is a new model, built upon the social model but incorporating elements of the medical model. It echoes the ICF perspectives on disability. It accepts that impairments identified by the latter are significant, but stipulates that far more problems are created for disabled people by social and environmental causes. Not all problems of impairment can currently be addressed, but if we recognise our environment as discriminatory we can do much to change it so that disabled people are enabled to higher achievement (Barnes and Mercer 2001, Bickenbach 2001, WHO 2002).

Unlike the social model, the social adapted model recognises that the inability of some disabled people to adapt to the demands of society may be a contributory factor to their condition. However, it still maintains that disability stems primarily from a social and environmental failure to account for and to provide adjustments for the needs of disabled citizens. The advantage of this model is that it does not concentrate on individuals' limitations, but takes account of people's capabilities and potential.

## The recovery model

Psychosocial recovery, or the recovery model, refers to the process of recovery from mental disorder or substance dependence, and/or from being labelled in those terms. Recovery has been defined as 'an individual's journey of healing and transformation to live a meaningful life in a community of his or her choice while striving to achieve maximum human potential' (US Department of Health and Human Services 2005). It incorporates a philosophy of support, respect, empowerment, choice, hope and social inclusion. Originating in programmes to overcome substance dependency, the concept of recovery in mental health usage emerged from deinstitutionalisation resulting in more individuals living in community settings but there being a perceived failure to support full recovery or enable proper integration into the community in a meaningful manner. The recovery model is a form of social model of disability, in contrast to a medical model of disability, and may involve 'consumers' and 'survivors' of mental health services as well as mental health professionals (Altman 2001).

Application of recovery model concepts to psychiatric disorders is comparatively recent. By consensus, the main impetus for the development came from the consumer/survivor movement, a grassroots self-help and advocacy initiative, particularly within the United States during the late 1980s and early 1990s. Other similar approaches developed around the same time, without necessarily using the term 'recovery', in Italy, the Netherlands and the UK. Developments were fuelled by a number of long-term outcome studies of people with major mental illnesses covering populations from virtually every continent, including the landmark WHO cross-national studies from the 1970s and 1990s, showing unexpectedly high rates of what were termed 'complete recovery' (20–25%) and 'social recovery' (40–45%). The cumulative impact of personal stories or testimony of recovery has also been a powerful force behind the development of recovery approaches and policies (Altman 2001).

## The cultural model of Deafness

Both the medical model and the social model are seen, at the least, to be in conflict with, and, at the most, inapplicable to deafness when viewed from the cultural model of Deafness. The capitalisation of the 'D' is intentional and is used to denote the dominant and positive view in which many prelingually Deaf people hold deafness. Lower case 'd' is used in all other meanings (Meadow-Orlans and Erting 2000).

Deaf cultural values are at odds with the dismantling of the residential schools since they were considered the best possible environment, the highest quality of life, in which to acquire and enrich sign language fluency and pass on deaf cultural values that serve as tools and solutions to challenges in a predominantly hearing world. This view sharply contrasts with the social model of disability, which finds segregated schooling of disabled children in special residential schools unacceptable and prefers the all-inclusive environment of mainstream/neighbourhood schools. This view has prevailed in most countries to the point that almost all Deaf children attend mainstream/neighbourhood schools in the US and to an increasing degree in the UK also (Barnes and Mercer 2001, Bickenbach 2001, WHO 2002). For many Deaf people the preclusion from developing a strong Deaf identity can lead to mental health difficulties. Inclusion and participation rather than assimilation is the target (Kitson and Thacker 2000).

The cultural model of Deafness arises from, in the main, Deaf people themselves, especially prelingually deaf people whose primary language is the sign language of their nation or community, as well as their children, families, friends and other members of their social networks (Altman 2001, Barnes and Mercer 2001, Ladd 2003, Meadow-Orlans and Erting 2000).

Because there is a Deaf community with its own language and culture, there is a cultural frame in which to be Deaf is not to be disabled. On the contrary, it is an asset of and for the Deaf community to be Deaf in behaviour, values, knowledge and fluency in sign language. It is within this community, bonded by shared culture and language, that Deaf people find themselves both enabled and socially advantaged. The experience of a language minority amounts to a social disadvantage no more or less troubling than it would be for any language minority (Barnes and Mercer 2001, Ladd 2003).

In contrast to the medical model of deafness, the Deaf community, rather than embracing the view that deafness is a 'personal tragedy', sees all aspects of the deaf experience as positive.

# References

Albrecht GL, Seelman KD, Bury M (eds) (2001) *Handbook Of Disability Studies*. Sage Publications, California.

Allport GW (1954) *The Nature of Prejudice*. Addison-Wesley, Cambridge, Massachusetts.

Altman B (2001) Disability definitions, models, classification, schemes and applications. In: Albrecht GL, Seelman KD, Bury M (eds) (2001) *Handbook Of Disability Studies*. Sage Publications, California.

Barnes C, Mercer G (2001) Disability culture assimilation or inclusion. In: Albrecht GL, Seelman KD, Bury M (eds) (2001) *Handbook Of Disability Studies*. Sage Publications, California.

Braddock D, Parish S (2001) An institutional history of disability. In: Albrecht GL, Seelman KD, Bury M (eds) (2001) *Handbook Of Disability Studies*. Sage Publications, California.

Bickenbach J (2001) Disability human rights, law, and policy. In: Albrecht GL, Seelman KD, Bury M (eds) (2001) *Handbook Of Disability Studies*. Sage Publications, California.

Conway M (2000) *Investigation into the Development, Design and Ergonomic Suitability of the Mobile Hoist as a Transfer Aid within Domestic and Institutional Settings.* Unpublished, London Guildhall University.

Council of Europe (2006) *Council of Europe Action Plan (2006–2015). Report* to promote the rights and full participation of people with disabilities in society: improving the quality of life of people with disabilities in Europe. Council of Europe, Strasbourg.

Finkelstein V (1976) *Fundamental Principles of Disability*. Union of Physically Impaired Against Segregation (UPIAS), London.

Grieve J (2000) *Neuropsychology for Occupational Therapists: assessment of perception and cognition*, 2nd edn. Blackwell Science, Oxford.

Kitson N, Thacker A (2000) Adult Psychiatry. In: Hindley P, Kitson N (eds) *Mental Health and Deafness*. Whurr Publications, London.

Ladd P (2003) *Understanding Deaf Culture: in search of deafhood*. Multilingual Matters Ltd, Clevedon.

Meadow-Orlans K, Erting C (2000) Deaf people in society. In Hindley P, Kitson N (eds) *Mental Health and Deafness*. Whurr Publications, London.

Morris J (1991) *Pride Against Prejudice: transforming attitudes to disability*. The Women's Press, London.

Morris J (2003) Prejudice. In: Swain J, Finkelstein V, French S, Oliver M (eds) *Disabling Barriers – Enabling Environments*. Open University Press/Sage Publications, London.

Oliver M (1990) *The Politics of Disablement: critical texts in social work and the welfare state*. Macmillan Press, London.

Oliver M, Barnes C (2003) Discrimination, disability and welfare: from needs to rights. In: Swain J, Finkelstein V, French S, Oliver M (2003) *Disabling Barriers – Enabling Environments*. Open University Press/Sage Publications, London.

Popper K (1959) *The Logic of Scientific Discovery*. Routledge, New York.

Ratzka AD (1987) Report of the Second International Expert Seminar on Building Non-Handicapping Environments: Renewal of Inner Cities. Prague, October 15–17 1987. Independent Living Institute. Available at: www.independentliving.org/cib/cib-prague1.html (accessed November 2007).

Reynolds S, McDermid L (2007) *Position Statement on Welfare Reform*. The David Freud Paper and Social Firm Sector. Available at: www.socialfirms.co.uk.

Schoon-Eberly S (1988) Fairies and the folklore of disability: changelings, hybrids and the solitary fairy. *Folklore* **99(1)**, 58–77.

Seelman K (2001) Science and technology policy: is disability a missing factor? In: Albrecht GL, Seelman KD, Bury M (eds) *Handbook of Disability Studies*. Sage Publications, California.

Swain J, Finkelstein V, French S, Oliver M (2003) *Disabling Barriers – Enabling Environments*. Open University Press/Sage Publications, London.

US Department of Health and Human Services (2005) *Achieving the Promise: transforming mental health care in America*. New Freedom Commission on Mental Health, Rockville, Maryland.

Warner R (2006) An update on affirmative business or social firms for people with mental illness. *Psychiatric Services* **57(10)**, 1488–1492.

World Health Organization (1980) *Classification of Impairments, Disabilities and Handicaps*. World Health Organization, Geneva.

World Health Organization (2002) *Towards a Common Language for Functioning, Disability and Health. International Classification of Functioning, Disability and Health*. Available at: www.who.int/classification/icf.

Young M, Quinn E (1992) *Theories and Principles of Occupational Therapy*. Churchill Livingstone, New York.

# 4: Ecological conceptual practice models

In the previous chapter the overarching models that shape our perceptions of disability were described. Readers were given an understanding of the nature of models, their purpose and how a worldview is orientated and understood through using models. Occupational therapists and other professional disciplines require a strong theoretical foundation to support the credibility of their fields of endeavour, and the ability to explain the theoretical concepts that underpin their practice.

For some time there have been calls from many within the profession for the development of a unifying concept of occupational therapy (CAOT 1990, Chapparo and Ranka 1997, Kielhofner 1992, Stamm *et al*. 2006). The growing focus on theory and the development of models in occupational therapy has not followed a single school of thought or a single theorist, so a plethora of frames of reference and inconsistent professional language has been developed, adding to confusion surrounding the profession's use of such terms as 'paradigm', 'models of practice' and 'frames of reference'. To understand the nature of occupational therapy's theory and knowledge it is necessary to define these key terms before applying the knowledge to practice.

## Paradigms

Kielhofner (1992), drawing on the original work of Kuhn, posits that 'paradigm' may be defined as that knowledge which is fundamental to the profession, that which defines the nature and purpose of occupational therapy, giving wholeness and coherence to the entire profession. Paradigms are the accepted model or pattern through which we operate, organise and make sense of the world (Kuhn 1996). They are frameworks through which we see the world and in turn, how this constructed world shapes what we see. They emerge out of socially accepted ways of being and foster these ways of being to the exclusion of alternatives. Kuhn further defines a paradigm as: 'an entire constellation of beliefs, values and techniques, and so on, shared by the members of a given community' (Kuhn 1970, p.175). This definition appears in the 1969 postscript to Kuhn's original book, because originally the use of the term 'paradigm' was not clearly defined. The term remains imprecise due to the different uses it is given.

Since its understanding is broad it is therefore general and so paradigms do not provide a detailed or specific application for practice. Application to practice is, after all, not its purpose, which is to define the nature and purpose of occupational therapy, giving wholeness and coherence to the entire profession. The application to practice is detailed within frames of reference and approaches to intervention which will be discussed in Chapter 5.

Kielhofner (1995) proposes that the paradigm of occupational therapy consists of three components: the core assumptions, the focal viewpoint and the values of the profession. These three components consist of particular elements and centre on the profession's belief that occupation is essential to wellness and has a role as a restorative health measure; people's motivations and environments strongly influence their engagement in occupational performance. Kielhofner notes the early assumptions held by the profession and also shows how the paradigm began to shift from its early holistic focus to a second paradigm, one of a more reductionist and mechanistic focus during the mid to late 20th century with the loss of occupation as central to our unique understanding of health and wellness in humans. A third paradigm is emerging and this has returned occupation to its dominant, central position as core to the profession's knowledge base.

Occupational science is a relatively new and interdisciplinary field in the social and behavioural sciences, dedicated to the study of humans as occupational beings. The term 'occupation' refers to the goal-directed activities that characterise human time use over the span of each day and over the course of lifetimes. Occupational science was founded in 1989 by Yerxa at the University of Southern California, and was based on the earlier works of Mary Reilly. This understanding of 'occupation' is taken by many within the profession to be the core underlying philosophy of occupational therapy. In aspiring to restore individuals to health or to promote health, the occupational therapist uses knowledge from occupational science and the use of meaningful occupation in intervention. Put simply, occupational scientists *study* 'doing' whilst occupational therapists *enable* doing.

Occupation is defined as including everything that a human being does, such as physical, mental, social and rest occupations or occupations for productivity, leisure and self-care. Occupation is described as the relationship between the environment having a physical and a sociocultural dimension (occupational form) and the active doing of the individual (occupational performance). Occupational form is

**Table 4.1** Elements of an environment. (From CAOT 1997. Reproduced with the kind permission of the Canadian Association of Occupational Therapists.)

| | |
|---|---|
| **Cultural** | ethnic, racial, ceremonial and routine practices, based on ethos and value system of particular groups |
| **Institutional** | societal institutions and practices, including policies, decision-making processes, procedures, accessibility and other organizational practices. Includes economic components such as economic services, financial priorities, funding arrangements and employment support; legal components such as legal processes and legal services; and political components such as government-funded services, legislation and political practices |
| **Physical** | natural and built surroundings that consist of buildings, roads, gardens, vehicles for transportation, technology, weather, and other materials |
| **Social** | social priorities about all elements of the environment, patterns of relationships of people living in an organized community, social groupings based on common interests, values, attitudes and beliefs *Enabling Occupation: An Occupational Therapy Perspective, CAOT 1997* |

related to meaning, and occupational performance is linked to purpose. Occupational therapists consider meaningful activities of individuals as a contribution to health and apply these meaningful occupations in their treatment (Meyer 1977, Townsend and Brintnell 2002, Wilcock 1998, Yerxa *et al.* 1989). Additionally in this emerging paradigm the role of the individual's and of the occupation's context, including the environment, has increased in prominence as an enabling or disabling context for occupation (Bass-Haugen and Mathiowetz 1995, Christiansen and Baum 1991, 1997, Christiansen *et al.* 2005, Dunn *et al.* 1994, Kielhofner 1995, 1997, Law *et al.* 1996).

During the past 15–20 years, the role of the context including the environment has become central to all the evolving disability models (Altman 2001, WHO 2002). Concepts of interdependency and the impact of temporal features and of the environment (in its broadest sense – physical, social, cultural and institutional) on occupational performance in relation to disability has shifted the location of disability from being viewed as within an individual to a broader understanding of the term (Table 4.1). It is increasingly viewed as the experience of people with impairments within contexts that fail to adjust to or take into consideration their differing needs. As we have already seen in the previous chapter, the disability movement proposed the following as a definition of disability: 'the disadvantage or restriction of activity caused by a contemporary social organisation which takes little or no account of people who have . . . impairments and thus excludes them from the mainstream of social activities' (Finkelstein 1976). Prior to this time, disability was viewed as a pathology that could be medically managed and hopefully fixed. Such an approach fails to consider sufficiently the role of the environment as an enabler or disabler of occupational performance (Altman 2001).

The dominance of the medical model as the most appropriate way to view healthcare has been questioned by many disabled people; its relevance to their needs is not always apparent. The ascendancy of the social model of disability has found favour with many groups, occupational therapy amongst them. The emerging 'occupational' paradigm contains many of the values and beliefs supported by this model.

This is a good example of how overarching models can influence the development of professional practice. Indeed, the dominant medical model of the mid-20th century influenced the profession's development of the reductionist perspective and promoted a move away from the notion of occupation as central to the profession's core assumptions noted earlier in this chapter.

It may be seen from the above discussion that core knowledge can change over time within a paradigm but this is a slow process. Paradigms or core knowledge are protected by other knowledge structures that help to preserve a consistent view within a knowledge base. These structures are conceptual models, frames of reference and approaches to intervention. Simply put, the range and scope of theory that shapes and develops the profession may be understood as consisting of four levels (Neistadt and Crepeau 1998).

1. *Meta theory*: concerned with the meaning of occupation and its relationship with human health and wellbeing. It may be considered as being at the profession's core – its paradigm. It embraces such ideas as an integrated theory of occupational therapy and occupational science. This is the first level.
2. *Grand theory*: focuses on the wider goals and concepts capable of representing the broad scope of the domain of concern. Theory at this second level is captured within the construct of generic conceptual practice models such as the person-environment-occupation-performance (PEOP) model and model of human occupation (MoHO).
3. *Middle-range theories*: deal with a relatively broad range of concern but do not fully embrace the entire breadth of the professional domain of endeavour. This third level of theory relates to knowledge at the level of the frame of reference, such as the theory contained within physiological, psychological and behavioural primary frames of reference, each of which may be further subdivided

according to its particular orientation and perspective (Hagedorn 1995).

4. *Practice theory*: facilitates the therapist in applying the theoretical perspective which should in all cases be supported by available best evidence. This fourth level of theory relates to application and is more commonly known as the approach to intervention.

Meta theory has already been discussed in this chapter and the purpose and function of the remaining three will be presented later in this chapter and in the following chapter.

## Conceptual practice models

Conceptual models, also known as generic practice models since they can be applied to all fields of occupational therapy intervention, explain and link theoretical concepts to each other. Models may be described as a means to represent an aspect of the natural world in some familiar way so that our understanding of the complex element can be improved. A model is defined as a theoretical simplification of a complex reality and consists of several explicitly defined concepts. A concept is an idea or notion. Concepts are formed by combining particular characteristics of a thing. The notion that underpins the core assumptions of occupational therapy relates to the profession's understanding of occupation and how this impacts on health and wellness in humans.

In conceptual models, concepts form the basic building material. Conceptual models are schematic or graphic representations of concepts and assumptions that act as a guide for theory development. Thus, concepts form the basic structure of a theory. A theory explains phenomena by specifying which concepts or variables are related (Reed and Sanderson 1999). Some theorists divide occupational therapy models into three groups:

1. professional models that provide a wide description of the role and practice of occupational therapists;
2. delineation models that set boundaries and guidelines in terms of expected intervention for particular client groups, such as biomechanical, neurodevelopmental and behavioural models;
3. application models that describe specific assessment and intervention techniques (Neistadt and Crepeau 1998).

They argue that the three types of models identified can be organised in a hierarchy with the professional or practice model on the top, and conclude that the further development of occupational therapy models will involve a series of challenges for the profession to develop the definition of a generally accepted conceptual model (Neistadt and

Crepeau 1998). Indeed, what have been described as delineation and application models seem to better inhabit the realm of frame of reference and practice models or approaches to intervention (Reed 1998). These aspects will be considered later in this chapter.

Conceptual models that explain occupational performance have become a major focus of occupational therapy literature in the last two decades (Chapparo and Ranka 1997, Baum and Christiansen 2004). Occupational performance is defined as 'the result of a dynamic, interwoven relationship between persons, environment and occupation over a person's lifespan; the ability to choose, organise, and satisfactorily perform meaningful occupations that are culturally defined and age appropriate for looking after oneself, enjoying life, and contributing to the social and economic fabric of a community' (CAOT 1997, p.181).

Mosey (1981) referred to occupational performance as the domain of concern for occupational therapy. She described areas of human existence which were of most concern to occupational therapy as consisting of 'performance components within the context of age, occupational performance and the individual's environment'. In applying the 'view' which Mosey named a 'frame of reference' to practice in mental health, Mosey (1981) suggested that a person's overall quality of occupational performance depends in part on the balance established among the component performance, the environment and occupational performance. What is referred to as a frame of reference by Mosey is generally accepted as more closely resembling what the profession now views as a conceptual practice model (Chapparo and Ranka 1997, Kielhofner 2002).

The concept of occupational performance has become central to the development of models of occupational therapy. This process, which constitutes the doing of activities, tasks and roles, operates as a means of connecting the individual to roles and to the sociocultural environment (Reed and Sanderson 1999). Occupational performance is often graphically represented as a Venn diagram (Fig. 4.1). The shaded area illustrating the intersection of person, occupation and environment represents occupational performance. An enlarged shaded area indicates satisfactory occupational performance whilst a smaller shaded area represents unsatisfactory occupational performance (Baum and Christiansen 2004, Law et al. 1996).

Conceptual occupational therapy models are applied in practice by occupational therapists (Hagedorn 1995) and act as a guide to therapists and practitioners in shaping their worldview of the person and reinforcing the central paradigm of the profession which in the case of occupational therapy is the relationship between health and occupation. Practice models organise concepts and ideas held by a profession and evolve over time to reflect the growing and changing knowledge

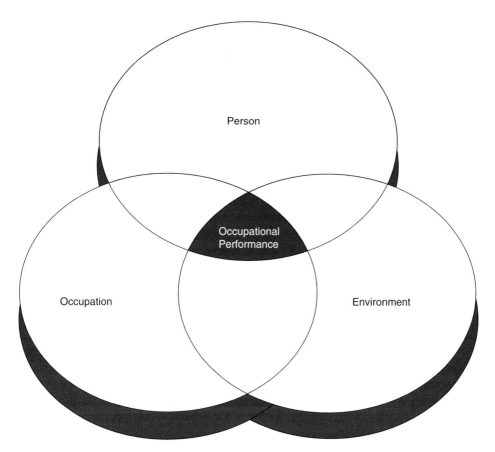

**Figure 4.1** Occupational performance. (From CAOT 1997. Reproduced with kind permission from the Canadian Association of Occupational Therapists.)

within a professional scope of concern; they provide a language by which practice can be labelled, terms defined and problems identified, thus leading to strategies for problem solving. They can also be a means of enlightening others within the multidisciplinary team (MDT) or practice setting about more inclusive practice measures.

As has already been noted, occupational therapists are often confronted with the context of overarching service delivery models in their daily practice and there may be tensions with implementing intervention from a solely occupational performance and essentially inclusive perspective with that of more dominant, reductionist views represented in some multidisciplinary settings. Such a collision course will undoubtedly provoke anxieties for the novice practitioner and pressures to conform will undoubtedly be encountered. The traditional 'medical model', which defines the individual as a passive receiver of medical care delivered by 'experts', is increasingly at odds with the occupational performance perspective which focuses on the choice of the person as core to its professional paradigm; other perspectives such as the recovery and social models are complementary to occupational therapy, having an inclusive paradigm at their core.

Practitioners must embrace the opportunities of working within and recognising the overarching service delivery models within which their practice is situated. Where these are incompatible with the perspective of occupational therapy, the practitioner's advocacy role becomes imperative in shaping the perspectives of their practice colleagues.

In the light of the changes within the overarching service delivery models, Baum and Christiansen (2004) identify six contemporary person-environment-occupation-performance (PEOP) conceptual practice models emerging in the occupational therapy literature. These models reflect the changing emphasis and understanding of disability and are in keeping with the core assumptions of the earliest occupational therapy paradigm mentioned previously in this chapter. The explicit and increased attention to the role of the environment as an enabler or disabler in achieving satisfactory occupational performance is a key focus within what is termed the emerging ecological conceptual practice models, so called because they all recognise the importance of the role the environment plays as it influences motivation, skills, roles and the relationship between humans and their environment.

Neither chronic illness nor ageing is well understood, leading to the possibility of a difficult social context for participants (Altman 2001). People with chronic illness emphasise wellbeing while health professionals emphasise symptom control. This leads to a possible dissonance between the two groups. It is with people from these groups (chronic impairment and ageing) that occupational therapists predominantly work.

In the 1960s Reilly (1962) succinctly identified the two key differences between occupational therapy and medicine – the latter's concern was with the prevention and reduction of illness whilst the former's concern was with prevention and reduction of incapacity resulting from illness. Reilly stressed the need to build a knowledge base from the point of view of the social sciences. Hence many of the profession's concepts emerged from the ideas of philosophy, psychology, social psychology, sociology and anthropology (Neistadt and Crepeau 1998). The dominance of predominantly ecological models in modern practice is therefore both heartening and not altogether surprising.

## Human ecology

In order to promote better understanding of what is meant by 'ecological models' within the discipline of occupational therapy, a brief overview of human ecology may be useful in clarifying the relationship with occupational therapy. Human ecology is an academic discipline that deals with the relationship between humans and their natural, created and social environments. Human ecology investigates how humans and human society interact with nature and with their environment.

Contemporary research in the field goes beyond the biological and economic foundations of human ecology to provide broader, cross-disciplinary perspectives on the ways in which human–environment relations are jointly influenced by physical, political, legal, psychological, cultural and societal forces. Such a broad view of environment echoes the occupational therapy interpretation of environment (Wasserman 2001).

Human ecology is an interdisciplinary applied field that uses a holistic approach to help people solve problems and enhance human potential within their near environments – their clothing, family, home and community. Human ecologists promote the wellbeing of individuals, families and communities through education, prevention and empowerment. Human ecology explores not only the influence of humans on their environment but also the influence of the environment on humans and their adaptive strategies as they come to understand those influences better. It is a way of thinking about the world and a context in which we define our questions, and provides ways in which to answer those questions (Wasserman 2001).

It is clear from the foregoing just how closely the field of occupational therapy echoes the concerns of human ecology. The key difference is that occupational therapy focuses on the 'doing' of humans and how that relates to health and wellbeing. However, the inderdisciplinary base of both disciplines is shared in many respects since the concern of both includes an interest in how the environment shapes and is shaped by humans in an attempt to achieve mastery, both are holistic and both strive to solve problems for individuals and enhance human potential within their near environments.

## Six ecological conceptual practice models

The six ecological conceptual models identified by Law *et al.* 2001 are listed below.

- Canadian Model of Occupational Performance (CMOP; Canadian Association of Occupational Therapists (CAOT) 1997).
- Person-environment-occupation model (PEO; Law *et al.* 1996).
- Occupational performance model (Australia) (OPM-A; Chapparo and Ranka 1997, Ranka and Chapparo 2006).

- The person-environment-occupation-performance model (PEOP; Christiansen and Baum 1991, 1997, Christiansen *et al.* 2005).
- The ecology of human performance model (EHP; Dunn *et al.* 1994).
- Model of human occupation (MoHO; Kielhofner 1995, 2002).

## Definition of key terms within generic conceptual practice models

### Person

A *person* is an individual with a unique configuration of abilities, experiences and sensorimotor, cognitive and psychosocial needs. Because of this uniqueness, precise predictability about their performance is impossible. The contextual variables and the meaning a task or occupation holds for an individual will strongly influence occupational performance (CAOT 1997, Dunn *et al.* 1994, Kielhofner 1995, 2002, Law *et al.* 1996).

### Occupation

This may be understood as an objective set of behaviours required to accomplish the goal. An infinite number of tasks exists for each individual and the roles inhabited by individuals, or demanded by the social functions of individuals, shape the individual's occupations (CAOT 1997, Dunn *et al.* 1994, Kielhofner 1995, 2002, Law *et al.* 1996).

### Context

The context is broader than merely the environment and although most generic conceptual practice models explicitly identify this as being solely the environment, some models such as the ecology of human performance (EHP) (Dunn *et al.* 1994) and the occupational performance model (Australia) (OPM-A) (Chapparo and Ranka 1997, Ranka and Chapparo 2006) specify that practitioners should consider temporal aspects as also being embodied within context. Individuals will determine temporal aspects dependent upon their needs and wants but temporal aspects may also be considered contextual because of the social and cultural meaning attached to them.

### Temporal aspects

1. *Chronological*: individual's age.
2. *Developmental*: stage or phase of maturation.
3. *Life cycle*: place in important life phases as socioculturally determined, such as career life cycle, parenting life cycle or educational process.

4. *Impairment status*: place in continuum of impairment such as acute-ness of injury, chronicity of impairment or terminal nature of illness (AOTA 1994).

## Environment

1. *Physical*: non-human aspects of context; includes the accessibility to and performance within environments having natural terrain, plants, animals, buildings, furniture, objects, tools or devices.
2. *Social*: availability and expectations of significant individuals, such as spouse, friends and caregivers; also includes larger social groups that are influential in establishing norms, role expectations and social routines.
3. *Cultural*: customs, beliefs, activity patterns, behaviour standards and expectations accepted by the society of which the individual is a member; includes political aspects such as laws that affect access to resources and affirm personal rights; also opportunities for educa-tion, employment and economic support (AOTA 1994, p.1054, CAOT 1997, Dunn *et al.* 1994, Kielhofner, 1995, 2002, Law *et al.* 1996).

## Occupational performance

Both the process and the outcome of an individual's interactions with the context and the requirements of the task are known as occupational performance. The performance range is therefore determined by the quality of the transactions between the person, the occupation and the context. The person–context transaction in task performance is the major variable that ultimately governs the performance range. Ecology, or the transaction between a person and the context, affects the task performance; task performance, in turn, affects the person, the context and the person–context transaction (Neistadt and Crepeau 1998).

Each of these models includes three central elements: person, occu-pation and context including environment. As implied by the models' names, they each acknowledge the transaction between the individu-al's occupation, the underlying performance components and the envi-ronment within which these elements meet. Where there is compatibility between these elements the outcome is satisfactory occupational per-formance. The reader is referred to the original sources for a detailed understanding of the application of these generic or conceptual practice models since such detailed discussion is beyond the scope of this text.

Common to each model, however, is the focus on enabling occupa-tional performance as fundamental to the health and wellness of the individual. The emphasis each model places on achieving this end varies in terms of the implied priority or dominance afforded to the primary action for change of each model or, to use an analogy, each model guides the practitioner through use of the model's lenses to view the concern from a particular stance within the overarching concepts of the model. The author suggests that for some this is demonstrated by the emphasis each model places on the components of the particular model. Common to all is the dominance of the person and their need to achieve satisfactory occupational performance as a central focus to each model in alignment with the profession's paradigm; the nature of the relationship between health and occupation.

However, the scope of application of each model then tends to place varying degrees of emphasis through its perspective on one or other of the three central components of the model. Some models provide very detailed information on the underlying performance components (including sensorimotor, cognitive, perceptual and affective/emotional components) of the person element that support occupational performance; this may indicate a rather reductionist or bottom-up overview of performance generally considered to be at odds with the more holistic or top-down perspective advocated by occupational therapy. Other models focus on the occupational roles and tasks that the individual wishes to achieve while still others guide the practitioner's focus to the environment and the supporting external context of the individual.

Some models, such as the PEOP, attempt to place equal emphasis on all three elements, postulating that the purpose of a conceptual practice model is to assist with understanding a phenomenon and not in the application of intervention. Implicit in this view is the holistic nature of occupational therapy and the applicability of the model across a broad spectrum of practice. This view acknowledges that a generic conceptual or practice model alone is not sufficient to guide practice (Barris and Kielhofner 1986). A practitioner needs to select specific theoretical frames of reference, related knowledge and approaches for intervention and use with a particular client's concern, using the conceptual practice model will guide the practitioner towards the most appropriate starting point – person, occupation or environment – or a combination of all three depending on the service user's need. This will be the focus of later sections in the following chapter.

### Model of human occupation (MoHO; Kielhofner 1995, 2002)

The MoHO, although an ecological model, is behavioural in focus (Stamm *et al.* 2006). The author acknowledges that although the model proposes occupational performance as its core and provides a powerful way to guide practice in the organisation and reorganisation of occupational behaviour, its focus is on the individual's routines and habits and on the individual as the key agent of change; motivation for activities must be determined as a requirement within this model (Law *et al.* 2001).

The centre of the MoHO is the human system. A system refers to any complex of elements that interact and together constitute a logical whole with a purpose of function. Occupational behaviour is a result of the interaction between human system, the task and the environment. The human system has three subsystems: the volition subsystem (for making occupational choices; consists of values, interests and personal causation), the habituation subsystem (consists of habits of occupational behaviour), and the mind-brain-body performance subsystem (describes the performance capacity). In addition, the environment influences human occupational behaviour: physical, social and cultural environments constitute occupational behaviour settings such as in the home, school or workplace and recreation sites (Kielhofner 1995).

Kjellberg and Haglund (1999) argue that the MoHO lacks the influence of the environment on human behaviour. The MoHO includes environmental factors and refers to such factors as 'press' and 'affordance' but has more emphasis on the person. It acknowledges the influence of environment but does not seek to explain the interaction and relationship between the person and the environment. The focus for change within this model is the individual and the environmental obligations for change in enabling occupational performance are less well defined. It is felt that the integration of the environment within this model requires strengthening (Brandt and Pope 1997, Kjellberg and Haglund 1999).

## Transactive ecological conceptual models

- Canadian model of occupational performance (CMOP; CAOT 1997).
- Person-environment-occupation model (PEO (Law *et al.* 1996).
- Occupational performance model (Australia) (OPM-A; Chapparo and Ranka 1997).

Although these models vary in terms of the emphasis placed on the process of implementing the model, each conceptualises occupational performance in broadly similar terms. Readers are referred to the original sources for more detailed discussion of these models. The models place equal emphasis on the three elements of occupational performance: the person, occupation and environment.

The OPM-A defines occupational performance as the 'ability to perceive, desire, recall, plan and carry out roles, routines, tasks and subtasks for the purpose of self-maintenance, productivity, leisure and rest in response to demands of the internal and/or external

environment' (Chapparo and Ranka 1997, p.58). It guides the practitioner to consider a detailed exploration of the core elements, subelements
and components of the model in determining the individual's occupational performance difficulty. It therefore directs the practitioner's
attention to related knowledge and frames of reference as the next step
in planning intervention.

The CMOP and PEO models define occupational performance as the
result of the dynamic relationship between the person, the environment and the occupation. They refer to the ability to choose and satisfactorily perform meaningful occupations that are culturally defined
and appropriate for looking after one's self, enjoying life and contributing to the social and economic fabric in the community. This is a particularly significant aspect of the CMOP and is the defining client-centred
core of this conceptual practice model. Occupations are groups of activities and tasks of everyday life (Townsend and Brintnell 2002, p.45).
The PEO model additionally recognises that environments, task
demands, activities and roles are dynamic and continually change and
shift throughout the lifespan. This model is placed in a developmental
context and guides the therapist/practitioner to consider temporal
factors when attempting to resolve occupational performance needs.
The temporal aspect of this model is represented in Figure 4.2. The
practitioner is guided to consider the scope of intervention in relation
to recovery, deteriorating condition and the needs of carers over time
where shared environments are a consideration.

### The person-environment-occupation-performance (PEOP) model

The PEOP model requires that information from disciplines outside
occupational therapy be sought, used, recognised and respected. The
complexity of human occupation, the uniqueness of individuals and
the diversity of environments make this necessary because no single
discipline is sufficiently broad to encompass the knowledge required
for all these areas. The subsequent chapters of this book present knowledge from fields outside OT and it will be imperative for practitioners
to acknowledge and embrace interdisciplinary information in client-
centred service delivery.

This model guides the practitioner's thinking and clinical reasoning
so that the broad scope of intervention can be considered. From an
occupational therapy perspective, the purpose of client-centred practice is to facilitate the health and function of the person whose occupational performance and participation are threatened or impaired and
to do this by drawing on relevant interdisciplinary information and
sharing this with the service user so that best outcome may be achieved
(Christiansen *et al.* 2005). The role of occupational therapy practitioners

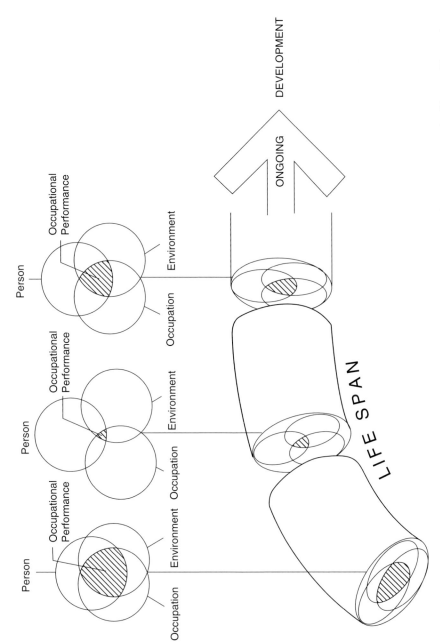

**Figure 4.2** Depiction of the person-environment-occupation model of occupational performance across the lifespan illustrating hypothetical changes in occupational performance at three different points in time. (From Law *et al*. 1996. Reproduced with kind permission from the Canadian Association of Occupational Therapists.)

is to help clients meet their goals for enhancing performance and reducing environmental barriers that limit their capacity to do what is important to them.

The PEOP model provides a framework to systematically understand and assist clients, whether individuals, families or organisations, to successfully meet their occupation-related goals (Fig. 4.3).

Because people, occupations and environments are complex and the relationships among them are dynamic, many performance issues may be understood as having several explanatory causes and will therefore benefit from multiple points of intervention. The practitioner may work with the client to identify opportunities for building personal capabilities, modifying environments or reconsidering occupational processes and goals. Each client, however, will have assets that may offset the problems that are interfering with occupational performance and participation (Christiansen et al. 2005).

During the past 10 years, the role of the environment has become central to all the evolving disability models. This is because the 'prevailing wisdom about the cause of disability has undergone profound change' (Brandt and Pope 1997, p.147). Prior to this time, disability was viewed as a pathology that could be medically managed and hopefully fixed. This approach excluded consideration of the environment. Recent approaches have viewed disability as the interaction between the characteristics of the individual (and his or her impairments) and the characteristics of the environment (Brandt and Pope 1997). The environment becomes important because it is thought of as being an active part of the individual person; just as glasses enable a person to see and a chair allows a person to sit, so a wheelchair enables a person to sit, to move, to socialise, to work and to be where he or she wants to be to do what he or she wants to do.

This change in approach has coincided with the further development of PEO models in occupational therapy (Bass-Haugen and Mathiowetz 1995, Christiansen and Baum 1991, 1997, Christiansen et al. 2005, Dunn et al. 1994, Kielhofner 1995, Law et al. 1996). These view occupation, the person (and his or her impairments) and the environment as the contextual elements that dynamically influence the meaningful activities, tasks and roles of daily life.

This change in focus does not mean that only environmental interventions are used. In fact, functional restoration remains central to all rehabilitation programmes. Functional restoration, however, is not the only approach used (Christiansen et al. 2005). What is critical for all professionals in the rehabilitation field is to 'understand the fundamental nature of the enabling–disabling processes. That is, how disabling conditions develop, progress, and reverse, and how biological, behavioural, and environmental factors can affect these transitions' (Brandt and Pope 1997, p.5).

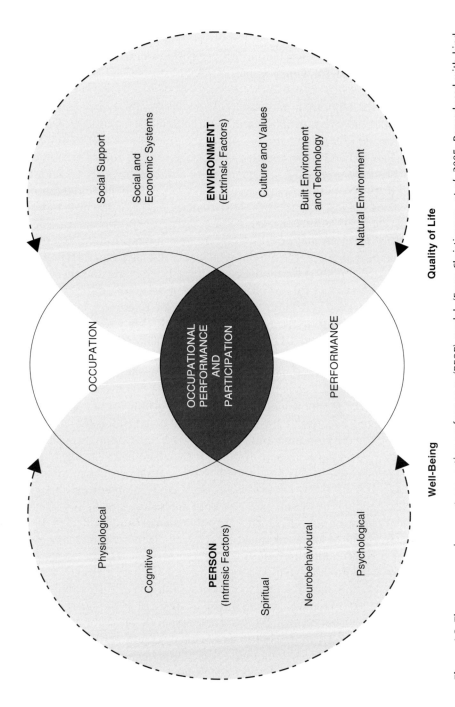

**Figure 4.3** The person-environment-occupation-performance (PEOP) model. (From Christiansen *et al.* 2005. Reproduced with kind permission from Slack Incorporated.)

Knowledge that supports our understanding of the impact of the environment in occupational performance will be discussed in detail in the following chapters.

### The ecology of human performance model (EHP)

The EHP model, whilst maintaining focus on the three core elements of occupational performance and occupational behaviour (Neistadt and Crepeau 1998), explicitly orientates the practitioner to the environmental context and its components at all stages of the process to suggest strategies for shaping the environment as a means towards achieving satisfactory occupational performance. Scholars within the field (Stamm *et al.* 2006) suggest that models that orientate the focus towards a particular element within the model are not true conceptual practice models of occupational performance, because an application to a particular aspect of practice is offered which may not have equal relevance to all occupational therapy practice settings. The generic and therefore necessary element of a conceptual practice model is missing. Stamm *et al.* (2006) suggest that 'approach' or 'frame of reference' may more appropriately describe the focus of this model. This view would also seem to be supported by Young and Quinn (1992) and Kielhofner (2002), when they suggest that in order for a model to be considered a conceptual practice model it must have generic applicability within the profession.

Yet the EHP model is well worth explicitly noting and exploring in greater detail because it guides the reader to consider the context including the environment and how it may be acted upon to facilitate satisfactory occupational performance. It therefore has a strong social model perspective and is one of the few conceptual practice models to consistently look to the context including the environment for change and reasonable adjustment as a means of achieving satisfactory occupational performance outcomes. Given the change in definition of disability from one of impairment to one in which disability is increasingly seen as a combination of both intrinsic and extrinsic factors or solely as a consequence of extrinsic environmental barriers (Altman 2001, Oliver 1990), this model seems to fit well with the World Health Organization's (2002) biopsychosocial model as detailed in the *International Classification of Functioning, Disability and Health* (ICF).

The social model of disability, as we have seen in earlier chapters, defines it as 'the disadvantage or restriction of activity caused by a contemporary social organisation which takes little or no account of people who have physical impairments and thus excludes them from the mainstream of social activities' (Altman 2001, p.103). A later definition proposes 'the loss or limitation of opportunities to take part in the normal life of the community on an equal level with others due to physical or social barriers' (Altman 2001, p.104). The EHP resonates with these definitions and suggests strategies to 'fix' the environment rather than the person in achieving satisfactory occupational performance. This model considers the naturalistic environment as fundamental to seeing the 'real' person and that true occupational performance can only be observed and experienced in the individual's natural context. It is the context including the environment that shapes, supports or inhibits an individual's occupational performance experience.

## Application

The primary theoretical postulate fundamental to the EHP framework is that ecology, or the transaction between the person and the context, affects human behaviour and task performance, and that performance can only be understood in context. The EHP offers a comprehensive framework for designing strategies (accommodations) to support occupational performance. This framework encourages individuals and disability specialists to consider not only the skills the individual might be able to develop, thereby focusing on the individual as the locus for change and adaptation, but also the skills the individual already has and ways to change tasks and contexts to facilitate successful performance.

The EHP does not assume that the individual must be 'fixed.' Rather, the focus (more than within the other five conceptual practice models) is on the transaction between the individual's skills and the resources of the context; any aspect that can be addressed to enable more satisfying performance is a viable strategy. Each transaction affects a person's future performance range and options, because the person, the context or the available performance range may be modified as necessary to achieve satisfactory occupational performance (Neistadt and Crepeau 1998). In some cases it will be the context that is the most amenable and appropriate domain to change. Very often it is in the person–context transaction where the greatest mismatch is experienced by service users.

In this model practitioners are encouraged to be concerned with the performance context as well as the performance demands. In particular, the notions that environments may offer opportunities for satisfactory occupational performance, known as *affordance*, or conversely that they can offer restrictions to occupational performance, known as *press*, are understood and applied within this model's perspective. Such notions are well aligned with the beliefs underpinning social inclusion theory and are strongly advocated by disability activists across all fields in both mental and physical health. The factors of affordance and press will be discussed in detail in the following chapter.

The key assumptions of the EHP model are identified as follows.

1. Persons and their contexts are unique and dynamic.
2. Contrived contexts are different from natural contexts.
3. Occupational therapy practice involves promoting self-determination and inclusion of persons with impairments in all contexts.
4. Independence and interdependence include using contextual supports to meet individual wants and needs (Dunn *et al.* 1994).

Five accommodation/strategy categories are offered for addressing individuals' needs and these are detailed below in relation to a service user with learning or mental health impairment.

1. *Establish/restore a person's abilities to perform in context.* This strategy addresses an individual's abilities. Here, strategies are designed to take advantage of strengths while working on performance skills that are weak and keep the person from achieving desired outcomes. This strategy therefore targets the person in their naturalistic context and the desired outcome is improved performance through renewed skill or ability.
2. *Modify/adapt contextual features and task demands so they support performance in context.* This strategy addresses features of the context and the task so they support the person's performance. These strategies build on the person's strengths and needs so weak areas do not interfere with performance. For example, if the client has poor memory, the practitioner might suggest environmental cueing and task simplification. This strategy does not fix the memory problem but reduces its influence on performance.
3. *Alter actual (naturalistic) context or task in which people perform.* The 'alter' strategies address the possible need to find an optimal context for the client. This means the practitioner and client acknowledge the client's skills and needs as well as the natural features of various contexts and search to find the best possible match between the two. Social firms mentioned in Chapter 3 relate to this strategy. By identifying a context in which the demands of the environment and the task match the service user's cognitive processing skills, rather than changing the existing environment (open employment) to accommodate the service user's needs, the service user is supported in completing the task (Dunn *et al.* 1994, Reynolds and McDermid 2007, Warner 2006).
4. *Prevent the occurrence or evolution of malpractice performance in context.* This addresses the ability to anticipate a problem in the future if no changes are made in the current pattern of living. When using this strategy practitioners are predicting likely negative outcomes that may impact on occupational performance in the future unless intervention is offered to mitigate this occurrence. The interventions may

address person, context, tasks singly or in combination, depending on the service user's need.

5. *Create circumstances that promote more adaptable or complex performance in context.* This strategy is different from the others in that it is used to enhance performance for all people through the provision of experiences to enrich the context and the tasks for the benefit of all. The 'create' strategy does not assume that a disability is present or that a disability has the potential to interfere with performance. This strategy fits with concepts frequently associated with universal design which will be discussed in detail in Chapter 6. In the case of an educational setting, the instructor is in the role of the architect and designs the instruction and curriculum for the benefit of all. An example might be that an instructor provides note pages on a website that are accessible for all clients in the class.

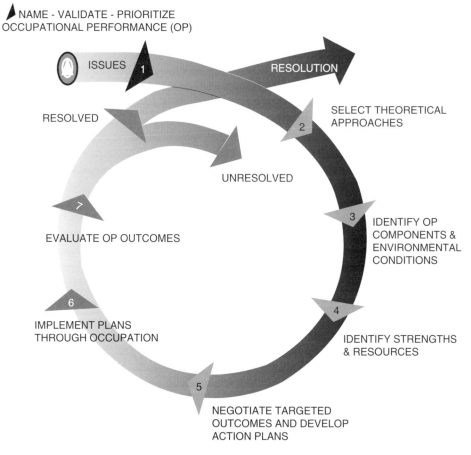

**Figure 4.4** Occupational performance process model. (From CAOT 1997. Reproduced with kind permission from the Canadian Association of Occupational Therapists.)

### Occupational performance process model

Increasingly the demands for greater interdisciplinary working and collaboration between professional groups place a burden on the practitioner to ensure that all relevant aspects from the interdisciplinary knowledge base have been considered in the intervention plan and delivery. One helpful way to structure information and points of action as practitioners progress through the occupational therapy process is to follow the Occupational Performance Process Model (Fig. 4.4). Briefly the model guides the practitioner through the occupational therapy process by means of seven stages. It is client centred and focuses on occupational performance. Readers are referred to the original source (CAOT 1997) for a more detailed account of the model.

## Conclusion

The ecological models presented in this chapter all focus on occupational performance as the central concern for occupational therapy. They also reflect the changing emphasis and understanding of disability and promote a deeper understanding of the person–environment transaction. Practitioners are encouraged to intervene at this level not as a last resort, when interventions at the level of the person have failed, but as an equal player in the intervention repertoire of the practitioner. The explicit and increased attention to the role of the environment as an enabler or disabler in achieving satisfactory occupational performance is a key focus within the emerging ecological conceptual practice models.

## References

Altman B (2001) Disability definitions, models, classification schemes, and applications. In: Albrecht G, Seelman KD, Bury M (eds) *Handbook of Disability Studies*. Sage Publications, California.

American Occupational Therapy Association (AOTA) (1994) Uniform terminology for occupational therapy, 3rd edn. *American Journal of Occupational Therapy* **48**, 1047–1054.

Barris R, Kielhofner G (1986) Beliefs, perspectives, and activities of psychosocial occupational therapy educators. *American Journal of Occupational Therapy* **40**, 535–541.

Bass-Haugen J, Mathiowetz V (1995) Contemporary taskoriented approach. In: Trombly CA (ed.) *Occupational Therapy for Physical Dysfunction*, 4th edn. Williams and Wilkins, Baltimore, Maryland.

Baum CM, Christiansen CH (2004) Person-environment-occupation-performance: a model for planning interventions for individuals, organizations, and populations. In: Christiansen CH, Baum CM, Bass-Haugen J (eds) *Occupational Therapy: performance, participation, and wellbeing*, 3rd edn. Slack Inc., Thorofare, New Jersey.

Brandt EN Jr, Pope AM (1997) *Enabling America. Assessing the role of rehabilitation science and engineers*. National Academy Press, Washington, DC.

Canadian Association of Occupational Therapists (CAOT) (1997) *Enabling Occupation: an occupational therapy perspective*. CAOT Publications, Ottawa, Canada.

Chapparo C, Ranka J (1997) *Occupational Performance Model (Australia), Monograph 1*. Total Print Control, Sydney, pp. 198–198.

Christiansen C, Baum CM (eds) (1991) *Occupational Therapy: overcoming human performance deficits*. Slack Incorporated, Thorofare, New Jersey.

Christiansen C, Baum CM (eds) (1997) *Occupational Therapy: enabling function and wellbeing*, 2nd edn. Slack Incorporated, Thorofare, New Jersey.

Christiansen CH, Baum CM, Bass Haugen J (2005) *Occupational Therapy: performance, participation, and wellbeing*, 3rd edn. Slack Incorporated, Thorofare, New Jersey.

Dunn W, Brown C, McGuigan A (1994) The ecology of human performance: a framework for considering the effect of context. *American Journal of Occupational Therapy* **48(7)**, 595–607.

Kielhofner G (1992) *Conceptual Foundations of Occupational Therapy*. FA Davis, Philadelphia.

Kielhofner G (1995) *A Model of Human Occupation: theory and application*, 2nd edn. Williams and Wilkins, Baltimore, Maryland.

Kielhofner G (1997) *Conceptual Foundations of Occupational Therapy*, 2nd edn. FA Davis, Philadelphia.

Kielhofner G (2002) *A Model of Human Occupation: theory and application*, 3rd edn. Lippincott Williams and Wilkins, Philadelphia.

Kjellberg A, Haglund L (1999) A critical analysis of the Model of Human Occupation. *Canadian Journal of Occupational Therapy* **66(2)**, 102–108.

Kuhn TS (1970) *The Structure of Scientific Revolutions*, 2nd edn. University of Chicago Press, Chicago, p.175.

Kuhn T (1996) *The Structure of Scientific* Revolutions, 3rd edn. University of Chicago Press, London.

Law M, Baum CM, Dunn W (2001) *Measuring Occupational Performance: supporting best practice in occupational therapy*. Slack Inc., Thorofare, New Jersey.

Law M, Cooper BA, Strong S, Stewart D, Rigby P, Letts L (1996) The Person-Environment-Occupation Model: a transactive approach to occupational performance. *Canadian Journal of Occupational Therapy* **63(1)**, 9–22.

Meyer A (1977) The philosophy of occupational therapy. *American Journal of Occupational Therapy* **31**, 639–642.

Mosey AC (1981) *Occupational Therapy: configuration of a profession*. Raven Press, New York.

Neistadt E, Crepeau E (eds) (1998) *Willard and Spackman's Occupational Therapy*, 9th edn. Lippincott Williams and Wilkins, Philadelphia.

Oliver M (1990) *The Politics of Disablement: critical texts in social work and the welfare state*. Macmillan Press, London.

Ranka J, Chapparo C (2006) Effects of information processing impairment on everyday tasks in people with AIDS dementia complex. Paper presented at the 18th Annual Australasian Society of HIV Medicine Conference, 11–14 October, Melbourne.

Reed K (1998) Theory and frame of reference. In: Neistadt E, Crepeau E (eds) *Willard and Spackman's Occupational Therapy*, 9th edn. Lippincott Williams and Wilkins, Philadelphia.

Reed KL, Sanderson S (1999) *Concepts of Occupational Therapy,* 4th edn. Williams and Wilkins, Philadelphia.

Reilly M (1962) Occupational therapy can be one of the great ideas of 20th century medicine. *American Journal of Occupational Therapy* **16**, 300–308.

Reynolds S, McDermid L (2007) Position Statement on Welfare Reform. The David Freud Paper and Social Firm Sector. Available at: www.socialfirms.co.uk.

Stamm T, Cieza A, Machold K, Smolen J, Stucki G (2006) Exploration of the link between conceptual occupational therapy models and the International Classification of Functioning, Disability and Health. *Australian Occupational Therapy Journal* **53**, 9–17.

Townsend E, Brintnell S (2002) The context of occupational therapy. In: Canadian Association of Occupational Therapists (eds) *Enabling Occupation: an occupational therapy perspective*, 2nd edn. CAOT Publications, Ottawa, Canada.

Warner R (2006) An update on affirmative business or social firms for people with mental illness. *Psychiatric Services* **57(10)**, 1488–1492.

Wasserman D (2001) Philosophical issues in the definition and social response to disability. In: Albrecht GL, Seelman KD, Bury M (eds) (2001) *Handbook of Disability Studies.* Sage Publications, California.

Wilcock AA (1998) *An Occupational Perspective of Health*. Slack Inc., New Jersey.

World Health Organization (2002) *Towards a Common Language for Functioning, Disability and Health. The International Classification of Functioning, Disability and Health.* Available at: www.who.int/classification/icf.

Yerxa EJ, Clarke F, Frank G *et al.* (1989) An introduction to occupational science, a foundation for occupational therapy for the 21st century. *Occupational Therapy in Health Care* **6**, 1–17.

Young M, Quinn E (1992) *Theories and Principles of Occupational Therapy*. Churchill Livingstone, New York.

# 5: Frames of reference and approaches supporting practice

On its own, a generic conceptual practice model is not sufficient to guide practice (Kielhofner *et al.* 1983). As we have seen in the foregoing discussion on conceptual practice models, such frameworks require an applied mechanism that addresses the detailed requirements of a service user's occupational performance needs. Such a mechanism may be referred to as a frame of reference (FoR) which will in turn require a further detailed processing, known as an approach to intervention, so that the knowledge can be applied to a particular individual's needs in the practice setting, before the practitioner can implement therapeutic intervention.

An occupational therapist needs to select specific theoretical frames of reference and approaches for use with particular clients that draw on the broad interdisciplinary related knowledge that supports occupational therapy intervention.

Frames of reference can be seen to relate more to the field's interpretation of the related knowledge that occupational therapists draw upon in their practice and how they then integrate and align this knowledge with that of conceptual practice models; the way in which the therapist applies this knowledge in practice may be seen as the approach to intervention (Neistadt and Crepeau 1998, Young and Quinn 1992).

An important aspect of a conceptual practice model in occupational therapy is the underlying frame of reference. The frame of reference is based on philosophy or a paradigm and attempts to describe or explain what we believe or value. Thus, the frame of reference reflects viewpoints, beliefs or values.

## What is a frame of reference?

A frame of reference is defined as:

- a set of ideas, as in a philosophical or religious doctrine, in terms of which other ideas are interpreted or assigned meaning
- the particular angle from which something is considered.

The concept of a frame of reference is not all that complicated. It's a beautiful vase of flowers! The only difference is that the vase is created by someone observing it. When a given person looks at something, perceptual filters are used. Those filters are creative. They are created by the observer. What is created is a perception that is not exactly the same as the thing being observed. People look, then analyse. The analysis creates not another vase of flowers inside the mind but rather a perception of that vase of flowers. Thereby, the mind's eye sees not the vase of flowers but rather a perception of it. The two are not identical. The difference is essential and profound (Gale Group 2007, Young and Quinn 1992).

Therefore, a frame of reference is a specific kind of boundary created by the observer around a set of elements in interaction and this third definition most closely relates to occupational therapy's understanding of the concept.

- A set of ideas, conditions or assumptions that determine how something will be approached, perceived or understood.
- A set of interrelated internally consistent concepts, definitions and postulates that provide a systematic description of, and prescription for, a practitioner's interaction with a particular aspect of a profession's domain of concern (Mosey 1981).

There is an old story from India that aptly illustrates how frames of reference affect an understanding of phenomena. The story tells of six blind men who were presented to an elephant, a thing they had never encountered before, and each was required to explain what he thought the elephant was. The first man felt the elephant's side, and he thought that the elephant was like a wall. The second blind man touched its tusk, and was certain that the elephant was a hard, spear-like structure. The third caught hold of the elephant's trunk, and stated that an elephant was like a large snake. The fourth man touched the elephant's legs, and was convinced that the elephant was like a tree trunk. Yet a fifth man, after feeling its tail, thought that the elephant was similar to a frayed piece of rope. The sixth and last blind man felt the elephant's flapping ear and proclaimed that the elephant was a type of living fan.

The blind men went back to their villages and began teaching the people about the 'elephant'. Each founded his own particular school of elephant teachings and soon there were six different schools of thought regarding the elephant. Students and disciples of the differing schools would argue with one another, the snake school of thought competing with devotees of the fan doctrine, the rope philosophy in conflict with the tusk school, and so on. A seventh blind man, much older and wiser than the others, visited the elephant after the other six. The seventh blind man had taken the time to stay with the elephant, to walk all around it, to smell it, to feed it, and to listen to the sounds it made. He was the only person who was not convinced that he knew exactly what an elephant was like (Gale Group 2007).

## Understanding frames of reference

The story of the blind men and the elephant illustrates how an understanding of a phenomenon can be developed. This analogy can be applied to the learning within a range of disciplines and within disciplines.

Packages of closely related theory are known as primary frames of reference (PFR) (Hagedorn 1995). Frames of reference as used by occupational therapists explain a particular aspect of knowledge and can be put into four categories.

1. *Physiological:* we need to understand the body systems, such as the musculoskeletal, cardiovascular, respiratory and central nervous systems that support biological survival. Examples of therapy approaches (which refers to the way in which theoretical/scientific knowledge is applied in practice) supported by this PFR are biomechanical, rehabilitative and neurophysiological (known as neurodevelopmental in paediatrics and in the treatment of some neurological conditions such as stroke and traumatic head injury). These in turn apply the understanding from their viewpoint to the practice setting by use of applied approaches to practice. Approaches such as the remedial approach, adaptive approach, movement science approach (motor relearning), Bobath concept and conductive education are examples of approaches drawn from this particular frame of reference.

2. *Psychological:* we need to understand human development, how mental processes influence emotion and behaviour, how individuals learn and use cognition, and how identity and roles are established. Humanism, as a psychological theory, is reflected in client-centred therapy approaches and fits well with the overarching service delivery models such as the social model of disability and recovery model. Other theories are evident in behavioural and cognitive therapy approaches and draw on theories from the fields of behaviourism as a primary theoretical foundation.

3. *Educational:* this reflects theories that explore how individuals respond to change, acquire new skills and develop culturally appropriate values. This will influence learning styles and problem solving, and links closely with the psychological PFR, which reflects the developmental and hierarchical aspects of learning.

4. *Environmental*: this PFR has not been explicitly noted within the occupational therapy canon until now. Because of advances in medical science, people are living longer, many with chronic conditions. Neither chronic impairment nor ageing is well understood, leading to the possibility of a difficult social context for participants. People with chronic illness emphasise wellbeing. Health professionals emphasise symptom control. This leads to a possible discord between the two groups if knowledge from a symptom control view point is the only one used in practice. It is with people from these groups (chronic impairment and ageing), as noted earlier in this text, that occupational therapists predominantly work. These people have the greatest need for the context including the environment to adjust their demands to match the abilities of this population. Therefore an environmental PFR should reflect theory that explores how the environment impacts on the occupational performance levels and perceived wellbeing of individuals.

There are numerous frames of reference that guide a practitioner's intervention within a domain of concern. Formerly, by following medicine's lead, occupational therapy defined the effect of a client's engagement in activity in narrow terms based on biomedical and psychoanalytical knowledge (Neistadt and Crepeau 1998). Since the purposes of occupational therapy and medicine are different, it therefore follows that their guiding knowledge should also reflect these differences. In the 1960s Reilly (1962) urged the profession to build a knowledge base that illuminated understanding about occupation and its influence on human welfare from the point of view of the social sciences (Neistadt and Crepeau 1998).

The perspective of many of the FoRs on which occupational therapy draws derives from the medical and psychoanalytic worldview to a greater or lesser extent. The focus of this worldview is to address (prevent and or cure) 'illness' rather than promote wellbeing and quality of life issues for those with chronic conditions or those undergoing the natural ageing process (although these outcomes may be byproducts of that intervention) and thus it provides a predominantly reductionist orientation to intervention. Practitioners are encouraged to actively consider the role of the broad environment to enhance their understanding of factors that impact on the occupational performance levels of clients. By altering an element within the environment (natural/physical, built, social, cultural, institutional and political) impediments to occupational performance for many of our clients may diminish significantly. From the previous chapter it is clear that an application of a guiding conceptual practice model is necessary in practice so that therapy can be organised in a way that is compatible with the ethos of the profession. Balancing the reductionist perspective of much of the related knowledge from other fields that practitioners utilise during the occupational therapy process against knowledge from the fields of design, ergonomics, ecology and environmental psychology will therefore provide a broad knowledge range to guide intervention.

## The environmental adjustment frame of reference

The interdisciplinary knowledge presented below underpins the view of the environmental adjustment FoR (see Fig. 5.1). The worldview is that of the person–context including the environment transaction. Responding to Reilly's urge from the 1960s, it derives from an interdisciplinary knowledge base drawing on the fields of design, ergonomics, psychology, ecology and the social sciences. The FoR deliberately chooses not to align itself with the reductionist connotations associated with the term 'adaptation' and has opted instead for a more explicit alignment with the universal design perspective.

> 'In considering the current definition of universal design, perhaps the term "adaptation" itself should be removed or fully explained. Adaptation is unacceptable as a means to universal design if common understandings of the term are used: reconstruction, renovation, or remodeling. This implies a good deal of effort and cost. However, designing for simple and low effort alterations (more like the idea of adjustability) maybe an acceptable route to a universal outcome' (Duncan 2007, p.22).

### The significance of perceived control

A review of the literature revealed perceived control to be highly significant in relation to wellbeing. The nervous system of human beings reacts not to stimulation but to change in stimulation (Kielhofner 1978, Lawton 1980, Norman 1999, Pheasant 1996, Reilly 1962, Wilcock 2001). Studies demonstrate that the removal of environmental stimulation results in disordered thoughts and behaviour. Humans need something to work against to balance them – a challenge (Lawton 1980).The literature shows that human interaction with the environment is a purposeful challenge. In order to *do* something, people need to interact with their environment. Furthermore, in order to achieve their goals they need to *control* that interaction. To this end, people use a wide range of abilities and skills to respond to and manipulate a range of environments in subtle and sophisticated ways.

Although people with a high level of skill in one or two areas, but not in others, might control the environments to which they are suited in a highly effective manner, they have greater difficulty in environments that do not match their skills (Gibson 1977, 1979, Lawton 1980). Those with few skills might only be able to respond in basic and relatively ineffective ways. In relation to a sense of wellbeing, it is the *perception* of environmental control that appears to be important. Later in this section we will see how Norman's (1999) definition of the concept of affordance, the usability of one's environment, also views the user's perception of acting on the environment as being crucial to a sense of wellbeing or having satisfactory occupational performance outcomes.

This *perception* has an impact not only on wellbeing but also upon survival. Perceived failure of control in a personally significant context can lead to a phenomenon that is described as *learned helplessness*. Such a person appears to lose all confidence in being able to effect environmental change or meet personal needs. Some of the negative effects of learned helplessness are boredom, reduced activity, passivity and depression (Lawton 1980). It is likely that when individuals feel able to practise some level of autonomy and choice they will feel happier and be more active than individuals who perceive that their occupational role performance has been absorbed or assumed by their carers or partners.

### The significance of perceived control – summary

- Humans function in terms of their environmental interaction.
- Sense of wellbeing is subjective rather than objective.
- Control of environmental interaction is central to wellbeing.
- Loss of perceptions of control can shorten life (Lawton 1980).

### Environmental interaction and perceived control

Maslow theorised that humans work towards an ultimate goal of self-actualisation by fulfilling their needs (Kielhohner 1995, Neistadt and Crepeau 1998). A simplified version of Maslow's hierarchy proposes four levels of need from lowest to highest: physiological/health needs, emotional/personal needs, participation and extrapersonal needs, and life satisfaction and esteem needs. Maslow's view was based upon the person's perception of self and environment, and therefore his hierarchy related to what was perceived as personally meaningful at any given moment.

Maslow mentions a number of constructs related to a sense of control; for example, it was thought there was an inherent satisfaction in influencing the environment successfully which engenders what is called a 'feeling of efficacy'. He theorised that this in turn gives humans a feeling of self-esteem, and that high or low self-esteem is related to their sense of confidence, based on experience, that they are environmentally competent.

Bandura (1977, 1982) further developed the concept and termed it self-efficacy. He defined efficacy as a generative capability in which cognitive, social, emotional and behavioural skills are organised and effectively orchestrated to serve innumerable purposes. The concept of self-efficacy is an important component of the volitional subsystem within the MoHO (Keilhofner 1995). He defined perceived self-efficacy as what a person believes they can do with what they have under a variety of circumstances. A large body of research has been developed around the construct of self-efficacy. Participation is always influenced by the characteristics of the environment in which it occurs.

Through a process known as arousal, environments can influence our desire to interact with or explore our environment. Arousal has both physiological as well as psychological characteristics related to one's level of alertness and has its most obvious effect on performance when people are bored and inattentive (underaroused) or anxious (overaroused). The degree of match between the characteristics of the environment and a person's capacities, interests and values may influence the desire to explore or interact within that setting. Calkins *et al.* (2001) note that the characteristics of settings that influence arousal must be carefully considered, so that an optimal level (producing neither boredom nor anxiety) is attained. Service users confined within some hospital settings frequently report experiencing boredom. Very often this is due to environmental–ability mismatch. Practitioners are charged with identifying the 'just right' challenge for service users so that optimal levels of arousal can be facilitated and sustained. Periods of hospitalisation should offer service users the opportunity to develop occupational performance skills in addition to receiving medical intervention. By developing a deep awareness of the person–environment transaction, occupational therapists have much to offer in the design and delivery of enriched environments that facilitate and stimulate satisfactory occupational performance outcomes for service users.

## Environmental affordance

Whether or not individuals believe they can act effectively in their world will also be determined by the actuality of their context. The structure and resources available within their near and extended environments will provide the platform for successful person–environment transactions.

James Jerome Gibson, an American psychologist, is considered one of the most important 20th-century scientists in the field of visual perception. In his classic work *The Perception of the Visual World* (1977) he rejected the fashionable behaviourism for a view based on his own experimental work, which pioneered the idea that animals 'sampled' information from the 'ambient' outside world. He also coined the term 'affordance', meaning the interactive possibilities or 'fit' of a particular object or environment. This concept has been extremely influential in the field of design and ergonomics and must be embraced and understood by the practitioner when determining whether limitations or opportunities at the level of the person–environment transaction need to be addressed so that the occupational performance of individuals can be influenced.

In his later work (*The Ecological Approach to Visual Perception*, 1979), Gibson became more philosophical and criticised cognitivism in the same way he had attacked behaviourism. Gibson argued strongly in favour of 'direct perception', or 'direct realism', as opposed to cognitivist 'indirect realism'. He termed his new approach 'ecological psychology'. He explained affordances as all action possibilities latent in the environment, objectively measurable and independent of the individual's ability to recognise them, but always in relation to the individual and therefore dependent on their capabilities (Gibson 1977, 1979). For instance, a narrow rope bridge spanning a stream does not afford the act of cycling or the act of propelling a wheelchair or the act of a parent pushing a child in a wheeled buggy. Applying this view to those with chronic mental health impairment with consequent difficulty in cognitive processing and/or associated affective difficulties may make it clear that environments with poor signage and complex information are too demanding or offer poor 'affordance' for their particular capabilities. This group may also be challenged by work environments demanding high productivity output coupled with low social support mechanisms, as seen in many competitive work environments. The affordances offered within many 'social firm' vocational settings acknowledge the capabilities of such populations. The affordance of the 'community' context provided within many social firms has led to the development of several successful enterprises across Europe and internationally, providing a 'supported' opportunity for employment (Reynolds and McDermid 2007).

In 1988, Donald Norman appropriated the term 'affordances' in the context of human–machine interaction to refer to just those action possibilities which are readily perceivable by an individual. It makes the concept dependent not only on the physical capabilities of the individual but also on their goals, plans, values, beliefs and past experience and so differs from Gibson's definition in this regard. If an individual steps into a room containing a chair and a table, Gibson's original definition of affordances allows that the individual may sit on the table and place a dinner plate on the chair, because that is objectively possible. Norman's definition of (perceived) affordances captures the likelihood that the individual will sit on the chair and place the dinner plate on the table, because of their past experience with these objects. Effectively, Norman's affordances 'suggest' how an object may be interacted with.

Affordance will, simply by observation, remind the user of similar items in size and occupational form. The user will know, either from conventions or experience, the functions of the task and the objects that enable the performance. Affordance can be misinterpreted if the user does not have the conventional knowledge. Therefore it is important for the practitioner, or designer, to study the user and consider whether the user differs from the designer with regard to the user's underlying capacities or performance components. Norman also points out the need for user interaction in the design process, where tests and feedback from the user should be used to improve the product or environment.

An affordance therefore can be understood to be an action that an individual can potentially perform in their environment. However, the more exact meaning depends on whether the word is used to refer to any such action possibility or only to those of which the actor is aware.

Norman's 1988 definition makes the concept of affordance relational, rather than subjective or objective. This he deemed an 'ecological approach' which is related to systems theoretic approaches in the natural and social sciences. The focus on perceived affordances is much more pertinent to practical design problems from a human factors/ergonomics approach, which may explain its widespread adoption. This will be discussed in Chapter 7.

## Gibson's affordances

- Action possibilities in the environment in relation to the action capabilities of an actor.
- Independent of the actor's experience, knowledge, culture or ability to perceive.
- Existence is binary – an affordance exists or it does not exist.

## Norman's affordances

- Perceived properties that may not actually exist.
- Suggestions or clues as to how to use the properties.
- Can be dependent on the experience, knowledge or culture of the actor.
- Can make an action difficult or easy.

According to Norman, the decisive factor is the perceptual information, so when it is there, regardless of whether the actual affordance also is, we may talk about a perceived affordance in Norman's sense of the term.

The distinction between Gibson's and Norman's sense of affordances allows us to distinguish between the utility/usefulness (Gibson) and the usability of an object (Norman). Designers design for usefulness by creating affordances (the possibilities for action in the design) that match the goals of the user (the relativity of the affordance vis-à-vis the user) and we improve the usability by designing the information that specifies the affordances (perceptual information). The two distinctions of the term should be considered by practitioners when determining with individuals their occupational performance needs. The objects and environments and the usability of such objects and environments required by individuals at the level of the person–environemnt transaction will be crucial in achieving enhanced occupational performance levels for users.

The concept of affordance has influenced architectural design and has powerful implications for the strategies occupational therapists can use to influence occupation-related performance and meaning.

## Environmental press

The personality theorist Murray (Calkins *et al.* 2001, Zeisel 2001) was one of the first to recognise in 1938 that characteristics of places influence behaviour by creating demands or expectations for behaviour, either objectively or as subjectively perceived by the individual. His term for this phenomenon was *press*. The idea that places influence activities and meanings has been refined and extended by other investigators, including Lawton (1980), and has been given prominence in the occupational therapy literature by Barris and colleagues (Barris 1985, Hamilton 2003, Rowles 1991).

Lawton (1980) provided insight into the processes determining whether environmental interactions were deemed successful or unsuccessful by the person and proposed an ecological model of ageing. This model utilised the concepts of environmental competence and environmental press. Lawton and others viewed competence as a characteristic of the person, while environmental press represented a demand, with some motivating quality, that is placed upon the person by the environment. Environmental press might be objective, or construed by the person, but it is a demand that is relevant and specific to a need of the person (Barris 1985).

To take a simple example, many railway stations in the UK and elsewhere have daunting flights of steps (an objective environmental press) to the railway platform. If a person wishes to catch a train, then negotiating these steps becomes a demand construed by the person (a subjective environmental press). It must be met in order to achieve the desired goal of catching a train. If the person is still fully mobile, (s)he is *competent* to meet this demand. If the person has problems with mobility, then the environmental demand might be too great, leading to an inability to carry out the activity that required catching a train. Thus Lawton (1980) talked about the person–environment transaction and described the outcome of such transactions in terms of occupational behaviour.

Lawton and Nahemow (1979) developed the press–competence model, depicted as a continuum of competence on one axis while a continuum of environmental press formed the other. The model has the advantage of linking behaviour to environmental press and competence. Behaviour in the model is considered as adaptive through to maladaptive in relation to both competence and environmental press, with a corresponding affective response. Where competence is low and environmental press is high, then behaviour is adaptive and the affective response is negative. When the environment offers little or no challenge to a highly competent person, the affective response is likewise negative. In the middle of the model sits the adaptation level. This was defined by Lawton (1980) as representing '. . . a state of balance between the level of external stimulation and the sensitivity of the person's sensory, perceptual and cognitive state' (p.45). A person at the adaptation level tends to adapt to any given level of stimulation in such a way that awareness of the stimulation recedes (Lawton 1980). An example of this is the initial awareness of the ticking sound of a new clock or sound of a train passing close to one's home; these can be disruptive but over time the noise ceases to intrude. A change of intensity or change in the rhythm brings it back to awareness (Lawton 1980).

Each person has a different point at which they reach the adaptation level for a given environmental stimulus because all humans have differing competencies (Lawton 1980). Lawton suggested that the zone of maximum comfort was where people feel relaxed and a bit understimulated. The person may feel bored but not excessively so. The zone of maximum performance potential provides sufficient stimulation to make people want to respond to it. In this zone people perceive competence to a level where they feel challenged and are able to meet personal and environmental demands, experiencing interest and pleasure (Lawton 1980).

The press–competence model (Lawton and Nahemow 1979) provides some insight into how a sense of control might be perceived differently by different people with differing needs and competencies functioning in differing environments. Taking mobility in older people as an example, perhaps individuals may find that the familiar environment of home offers challenges that they can mostly meet, putting them in the adaptation zone or the zone of maximal performance potential in the press–competence model. The community environment may offer high levels of demand in relation to older people's competence, so that they may be represented in the zone of negative affect and maladaptive behaviour in the model, preferring the self-restriction of staying indoors.

The environmental docility hypothesis proposed by Lawton (1980) relates to this model. This hypothesis stated that people with low levels of environmental competence rely on the environment to support them much more than people with high levels of competence. It follows that older people or those with physical or psychological impairments might fit only within environments that support that need (Calkins *et al.* 2001) unless the wider community environment acknowledges the range of different individual competencies amongst individuals and adjusts the wider environment to take account of these differences (Duncan 2007). For example, someone using a walking frame can only match with an environment with steps and doorways of sufficient width and depth to allow passage, whereas those without a mobility disability can match a wider range of environments. Those with cognitive processing difficulties may experience press within environments that take little account of the way in which information is provided or how the ambient environmental conditions impact on such an individual's ability to participate (Calkins *et al.* 2001, Zeisel 2001).

The relevance of the focus of a FoR should be considered in the light of evolving knowledge. As we saw in earlier chapters, the changing perspectives within models of disability have profoundly influenced the development and context of care offered across a range of service settings. A shift to the community as the primary care setting for the majority of service users across a range of clinical groups is gathering momentum. We are beginning to see (in some cases) the positive impact the environment has on occupational performance for many service users although this experience is not universal – yet! The environment (natural/physical, social, cultural, institutional and political) is gradually adjusting to the demands of the disability activists. By enacting legislation to address the environmental limitations that face many disabled people a realisation is growing that the implicit benefits of appropriately designed, organised and delivered processes, objects and environments impact favourably on us all.

The environmental adjustment frame of reference, graphically illustrated in Figure 5.1, takes account of both individuals' capacities and the environmental context by identifying the elements within an environment that offer press or affordance to a particular individual in relation to their occupational performance needs and individual skill competence. It promotes the adjustment of the context of individuals as a means to facilitate greater participation on all levels, thereby achieving greater inclusion. This FoR is applied in practice through the

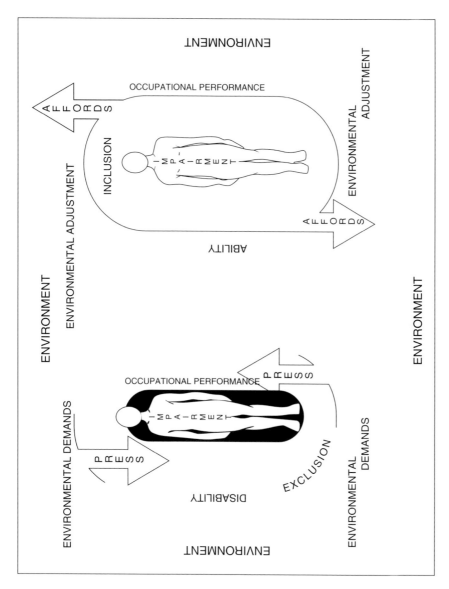

**Figure 5.1** Environmental adjustment frame of reference. (Drawn by Kasia Halota.)

universal design approach, the principles of which will be described in full in the following chapter.

The environmental adjustment frame of reference brings together related knowledge from an interdisciplinary base in guiding the practitioner towards selecting the most appropriate knowledge relating to the person–environment transaction aspect of occupational performance.

## Approaches to intervention

Approaches may be expressed as the means whereby the knowledge within frames of reference is implemented and applied in the practice setting. Many therapy approaches draw upon theory from more than one PFR. Theory can be thought of as reductionist (sometimes called mechanistic) or holistic. Neither is right nor wrong as they present contrasting ways of looking at knowledge.

The underlying theory of individual therapy approaches and models of practice has a tendency to be more or less reductionist or holistic. Consequently, it is important not to select a holistic conceptual model of practice and then use only reductionist FoRs within it. A practitioner may use many FoRs so that the best evidence-based knowledge is available to meet service users' needs.

To use therapy approaches successfully, we need to understand the underlying theory. Essentially all treatment approaches can be categorised under three headings; these are remedial, adjustment/adaptive and educational. It is beyond the scope of this text to discuss all treatment approaches in detail and the reader is referred to the original sources. However, one approach, that of universal design (adjustment), will be explored in greater detail in the following chapter. It is proposed that this approach is compatible for use with the environmental adjustment FoR described in this chapter.

## References

Bandura A (1977) Self-efficacy: toward a unifying theory of behavioural change. *Psychological Review* **84,** 191–215.

Bandura A (1982) Self-efficacy mechanisms in human agency. *American Psychologist* **37,** 122–147.

Barris R (1985) Environmental interactions: an extension of the model of occupation. *American Journal of Occupational Therapy* **36(10),** 637–644.

Calkins M, Sanford, J, Proffitt M (2001) Design for dementia: challenges and lessons for universal design. In: Preiser W, Ostroff E (eds) *Universal Design Handbook.* McGraw-Hill, New York.

Duncan R (2007) *Universal Design – Clarification and Development. A Report for the Ministry of the Environment.* Government of Norway, Oslo.

Gale Group (2007) Online Encyclopedia. Available at: http://infotrac.galegroup.com/default.

Gibson JJ (1977) The theory of affordances. In: Shaw R, Bransford J (eds) *Perceiving, Acting, and Knowing.* Erlbaum, Hillsdale, New Jersey.

Gibson JJ (1979) *The Ecological Approach to Visual Perception.* Houghton Mifflin, Boston, Massachusetts.

Hagedorn R (1995) *Occupational Therapy: perspectives and processes.* Churchill Livingstone, New York.

Hamilton TB (2003) Occupations and places. In: Christiansen C, Townsend E (eds) *Introduction to Occupation: the art and science of living.* Prentice-Hall, Upper Saddle River, New Jersey, pp.173–196.

Kielhofner G (1978) General system theory: implications for the theory and action in occupational therapy. *American Journal of Occupational Therapy* **32,** 637–645.

Kielhofner G (1995) *A Model of Human Occupation: theory and application,* 2nd edn. Williams and Wilkins, Baltimore, Maryland.

Kielhofner G, Barris R, Watts J (1983) *Psychosocial Occupational Therapy: practice in a pluralistic arena.* Ramsco, Laurel, Maryland.

Lawton MP (1980) *Environment and Aging.* Brooks-Cole, Monterey, California.

Lawton MP, Nahemow L (1979) Social areas and the well being of tenants in housing for the elderly. *Multivariate Behavioral Research* **14,** 463–484.

Mosey AC (1981) *Occupational Therapy: configuration of a profession.* Raven Press, New York.

Neistadt E, Crepeau E (eds) (1998) *Willard and Spackman's Occupational Therapy,* 9th edn. Lippincott Williams and Wilkins, Philadelphia.

Norman DA (1999) Affordances, conventions, and design. *Interactions* **6(3),** 38–41.

Pheasant ST (1996) *Body Space: anthropometry, ergonomics and the design of work,* 3rd edn. Taylor and Francis, London.

Reilly M (1962) Occupational therapy can be one of the great ideas of 20th century medicine. *American Journal of Occupational Therapy* **16,** 300–308.

Reynolds S, McDermid L (2007) Position Statement on Welfare Reform. The David Freud Paper and Social Firm Sector. Available at: www.socialfirms.co.uk.

Rowles GD (1991) Beyond performance: being in place as a component of occupational therapy. *American Journal of Occupational Therapy* **45(3),** 265–271.

Wilcock A (2001) *Occupation for Health Volume 1: a journey from self health to prescription.* Lavenham Press, Suffolk.

Young M, Quinn E (1992) *Theories and Principles of Occupational Therapy.* Churchill Livingstone, New York.

Zeisel J (2001) Universal design to support the brain and its development. In: Preiser W, Ostroff E (eds) *Universal Design Handbook.* McGraw-Hill, New York.

# PART 2
# Inclusive Design: Principles for Practice

'Several similar contests with the petty tyrants and marauders of the country followed, in all of which Theseus was victorious. One of these was called Procrustes or the stretcher. He had an iron bedstead on which he used to tie all travellers who fell into his hands. If they were shorter than the bed he stretched their limbs to make them fit; if they were longer than the bed he lopped off a portion' (Pheasant 1996, p.3).

# 6: Knowledge from the field of design

The opening lines of Stephen Pheasant's book *Body Space* are taken from *The Age of Fable* by Thomas Bullfinch (1796–1867) and serve well here also (see previous page).

For many of those disabled by the environment the Procrustean bedstead is an all too familiar reality. Most of us could recount times when we have encountered environments (built, physical and social) and artefacts that did not adequately meet our needs. Consider travelling by public transport or private vehicles, entering a busy reception area for the first time, seeking directions, encountering a PC with overloaded screen information, using the WC, having a bath, to name but a few. Consider both the physical and psychological demands of the task and the consequent effort required and fatigue experienced in its execution. For those among us without impairments in mind or body, functional use may be achieved by some adjustment and adaptation to a greater or lesser degree. However, there are many among us – the differently abled or disabled – for whom such adjustment and adaptation are supremely challenging, ineffective or impossible.

As we have already seen, theory serves a profession such as occupational therapy by providing answers to several major aspects related to distinctness and the integrity of the profession. One such area is that theory can be updated periodically to keep the knowledge base current with new knowledge and skills gained from working with other disciplines, and changes in the political, social and cultural perspectives. Occupational therapy is especially sensitive to changes in health-care delivery patterns (recovery and social inclusion) and politico-sociocultural trends (Reed 1998).

Developments within the fields of design and ergonomics coupled with subsequent policy and legislative changes and the growth of the ecological perspectives within the profession of occupational therapy allow for greater collaboration and interdisciplinary knowledge exchange towards achieving a more inclusive environment for all.

The impact of community care on housing design has become more apparent.

Many more people who need high levels of assistance now live in their own homes, instead of moving into residential care. Supplementary design guidance therefore needs to be developed to meet the needs of assisted wheelchair users and their carers. *The Manual Handling Operations Regulations* introduced in the UK in 1992 resulted in more scrutiny of the ergonomics of home design in promoting safety for carers and people with disabilities. A range of new lifting and handling equipment has been introduced into home settings, which now impacts on housing standards (Chapman 1999).

'Smart' technologies such as home automation, helplines and other forms of communication have evolved to address the needs of vulnerable people in their own homes. The full potential of technology in supporting care in home settings needs further research and evaluation (Calkins *et al.* 2001).

Universal design is influencing new-build housing design, through the use of selected design features such as level access and wider doorways to all new dwellings. These features make it easier for people with disabilities to visit neighbours and this promotes social inclusion. Beyond this, however, other adjustments are also needed to accommodate the psychosocial needs of many individuals with mental health difficulties who experience exclusion because of the way in which society is organised (Preiser and Ostroff 2001).

An inclusive approach to community needs also raises awareness about how housing design and the design of work can meet the requirements of people with visual or hearing impairments, mental health or learning difficulties, as well as people with restricted mobility. It is knowledge from the field of ergonomics and in particular from the branch known as cognitive ergonomics or human factors that is most helpful in promoting greater inclusion in these areas. The application and relevance of ergonomics will be discussed in greater detail in Chapter 7 (Pheasant 1996).

There is now a considerable amount of published design guidance available (BSI 2001, Chapman 1999, NDA 2002, ODPM 2006, Preiser and Ostroff 2001, Sangster 1997).This raises the question, 'What is best design practice?'. It is difficult to define what best practice is as it is constantly changing, driven by new technology, social change, legislation and advances in treatment and care. This chapter and the following are about how to achieve equality and inclusiveness for everybody in buildings and the external environment. They are also about how to ensure that everyone can make full use of the buildings and environments they live in, work in and visit. This means more than just an interpretation of laws or regulations.

The universal design perspective has evolved from just such an awareness and, as we will see, offers the practitioner a reliable and consistent way to approach design decisions ensuring the best evidence-based outcomes for service users.

The Center for Universal Design at North Carolina State University defines universal design as 'the design of all products and environments to be usable by people of all ages and abilities, to the greatest extent possible' (Orstroff 2001, Story 2001, p.10.3). For those of us involved in the fields of occupational therapy, design, architecture, ergonomics or any discipline concerned with how people use and are supported by environments and the artefacts within them, a challenge is placed before us: how can we consign the present-day Procrustean bedsteads to the realms of the past? Adopting an approach known as inclusive or universal design may be one way to achieve this.

## Housing Enabler tool

Before introducing the seven principles of universal design (UD) it is worth noting the shared history between UD and occupational therapy and how its influence is already firmly grounded in some areas of practice.

Occupational therapists (OTs) are facing increasing demands to demonstrate that their interventions are efficient and effective, including demands to use research-based methodology. Therefore there are increasing requirements on them to implement research findings and to demonstrate their application in practice (Fange *et al.* 2007). In spite of this, many OT interventions are still being implemented without the use of structured, research-based methodology.

At least one methodology exists, the Housing Enabler (HE), that supports practitioners in addressing the need for evidence-based practice in this area. Over several years a methodology for housing accessibility assessments based on the Enabler concept, i.e. the HE instrument, has been developed and optimised. The Enabler was developed in the 1980s by architect Ed Steinfeld initially for use by architects as a means to promote better usability in buildings. Uptake was low by this group but fortunately Swedish occupational therapists Iwarsson and Isacsson saw the potential to develop the instrument as a housing assessment tool for occupational therapists; hence the name change to Housing Enabler.

Steinfeld has long been associated with the universal design perspective and was one of the founding members of the principles of universal design (Story 2001). The congruence between occupational therapy and universal design is further illustrated in this background. The Enabler concept is based on the notion of person–environment (P–E) fit as described in the ecological theory of ageing and the relation of housing and health is closely linked to this notion. According to the docility hypothesis, individuals with lower competence are more sensitive to the demands of the environment than those with higher competence (Iwarsson *et al.* 2007, Lawton 1980, Lawton and Nahemow 1979).

The inter-rater reliability, as well as content and construct validity, of the HE have been developed through extensive research (demo version is available at www.enabler.nu for free download and is worth exploring). The HE instrument is complex and practitioners are required to attend a four-day assessment course comprising theory related to housing adjustment/adaptation and P–E fit and current housing provision policy, as well as teaching and practical training in HE administration (Iwarsson and Slaug 2001).

## Administration

The Housing Enabler instrument is administered in three steps. The first step is a combination of interview and observation, assessing functional limitations (13 items) and dependence on mobility devices (two items), i.e. the personal component of the concept accessibility. The second step is an assessment of physical environmental barriers, i.e. the environmental component of accessibility. This is based on a detailed observation assessing environmental barriers in the home and the immediate outdoor environment (188 items). The third step is the calculation of an accessibility score; for each environmental barrier item, the instrument comprises predefined severity ratings, operationalised as points quantifying the level of accessibility problems predicted to arise in each case. The severity scale is scored 1–4; higher points indicate more problems. In cases in which no functional limitations or dependence on mobility devices are present, the score is zero. On the basis of the assessments completed in steps 1 and 2, using special software the profile of functional limitations and dependence of mobility devices identified in each person is aligned with the environmental barriers identified. The sum of all the predefined points yields a score quantifying any accessibility problems present; higher scores mean more problems.

## Application

Based on experience and results from studies, Fange *et al.* (2007) concluded that a municipality or local government level database comprising HE assessments accomplished for individual housing assessments cases would have the potential to support housing provision and societal planning at municipality level. This tool also supports the universal design perspective and provides a very relevant assessment tool for practitioners.

## Universal design

### Definition

Universal design is the design of products and environments to be usable by all people, to the greatest extent possible, without the need for adaptation or specialised design. The intent of the universal design concept is to simplify life for everyone by making products, communications and the built environment more usable by more people at little or no extra cost. The universal design concept targets all people of all ages, sizes and abilities (Center for Universal Design 1997, Mace *et al.* 1991).

### The concept

A working group of architects, product designers and environmental design researchers has identified seven universal design principles for use in evaluating existing designs, guiding the design process and educating both designers and consumers about the characteristics of more usable products and environments.

The role of the occupational therapists as practitioners intervening at the level of the person–environment transaction embraces that of the designer when environmental adjustment is needed. The 'press' factors exerted by a given environment in interaction with an individual's capacities that may prevent satisfactory occupational performance come within the scope of OT practice. Hence there is a clear need for the occupational therapist to become fully conversant with a design approach that can be used to apply intervention within the environmental adjustment frame of reference introduced in the previous chapter (Center for Universal Design 1997).

Ron Mace, an architect, first used the term 'universal design' in 1985 when considering the usability of environments for a range of users. He was acutely aware of individual uniqueness and human diversity (Orstroff 2001). Living spaces have long been designed for use by one 'average' physical type – young, fit, male and adult. Yet only some of us fit that description and only at a particular point in the lifespan. As children, as older adults or as physically disabled people, millions are never average. Many millions more, because of a broken limb, serious illness or pregnancy, know how unsettling it is to try to function in an environment that no longer meets their needs.

In reality there is no 'average' that actually represents the majority because too many people have vastly differing requirements. The composition of our population is changing. Many people are surviving permanently disabling accidents and illness and even more are living longer. It would seem logical that the spaces built to accommodate this population must, by necessity, change also (Duncan 2007, NDA 2002).

Many inequalities and injustices of the past were built on the concept of the 'normal' person. To define one group in society as the norm, even a very large group, is to privilege that group and marginalise everybody else. In Chapter 2 we noted that society's response to dealing with difference was to marginalise by segregation those deemed to be different or deficient in some way. We no longer take this view and yet unless the environment adjusts to the range of diversity and needs of its inhabitants, continuing segregation and exclusion is the lived experience for many (DRC 2006).

Royal Mail (CEDC 2005) conducted a survey of medical retirement across its employees (some 180,000 people). It was found that many of those taking premature medical retirement were assessed by occupational therapists as being employable, but not within any of the workplaces available within the Royal Mail Group. Thus, because of the comparative inaccessibility of the work environment, the employees were being medically retired.

## Misunderstandings about disabled people

- People with disabilities don't go out much.
- People with disabilities don't want or need jobs.
- People with disabilities don't have families, marry or have children, so one-bedroom apartments should be sufficient.
- People with disabilities only need access to doctors' offices and other medical facilities.
- People with disabilities want to live together.
- People with disabilities are not affluent or self-sufficient, and thus are not an important part of the consumer market. (Mace *et al.* 1991)

A French television commercial shows able-bodied people trying to function and participate in a world designed for people with disabilities. Speaking persons approach receptionists, who respond only in sign language; a sighted individual looks for books in a library but finds them all printed in Braille; walkers slip down wet declines navigated by people in wheelchairs. A strong message is communicated: the world is harder when it is not conceived with your abilities in mind.

In the 21st century we recognise that people are all different. People change. Difference is a part of everyday life. As children we are small, weak and less aware. As we grow old we grow weaker, probably less aware and sometimes we even grow smaller. Any 'normal' society contains within it adult men and women, children, older people and people in all these groups with a wide range of diversity which for some means they are disabled by the organisation and structure of a disabling environment. Internationally, through the development of policy and law, we are moving to an ever more inclusive definition of what is normal, and are developing a greater understanding that the broad range of human diversity is central to this definition (WHO 2002).

There is a significant proportion of the population whose capacities, whether physical, intellectual or emotional, are impaired, temporarily or permanently. Impairment of the body or mind may change, limit or render impossible someone's ability to undertake a particular task. The environment can offer supports or obstacles (Duncan 2007).

Designers and other practitioners such as occupational therapists who are concerned with the practical day-to-day endeavours of humans need to appreciate the human diversity that exists within and outside a disability construct (Mace 1985).

Everyone possesses varying degrees of ability and disability so instead of viewing individuals as either able-bodied or disabled, other perspectives that reflect the temporal nature of all our characteristics – temporarily able-bodied, fully visual, etc. – may be more helpful. Perhaps a universal approach will help society move toward more inclusive considerations of the users of design (Duncan 2007).

> '. . . the concept of "functional accessibility" for specific groups, few in number, has started a trend toward universally designed solutions that benefit a wide range of people throughout their daily and life-long transitions' (Kochtitzky 2006, p.56).

Occupational science, the philosophy that underpins the core professional beliefs of occupational therapy, sees the concept of 'occupation' as referring to the goal-directed activities that characterise human time use over the span of each day and over the course of lifetimes (Yerxa *et al.* 1989). Given that humans are social beings, the bulk of our activity can be understood to embrace the concept of participation; participation that occurs within an environmental context with physical (built, climatic, natural), social and cultural elements. Therefore the congruity of the universal design philosophy with that of occupational science and occupational therapy is high since each is concerned with the person–environmant transaction and human action within that context.

When the inter-relationship between universal design and the *International Classification of Functioning* is considered, the relevance to the field of occupational therapy is further strengthened. Both the ICF and UD principles are based on similar underlying theoretical constructs. Both recognise the environment as a major influence on human experience and participation, and both recognise that people without impairments also experience limitations due to the influence of non-supportive environments (Steinfeld and Danford 2006, WHO 2002).

## Evolution and policy

User-focused design is not new; examples of user-tailored or human-centric design extend back thousands of years and often focus on occupational issues such as tools adapted to certain tasks (Duncan 2007). Roman chariots were built to the scale of warriors and the historic use of the dimensional term 'foot' gives evidence of our attention to the human form (Umbach 2006).

The architectural trends of the late 19th and early 20th centuries toward modernist and functionalist design seemed to consider the day-to-day needs of individuals. Architects such as Klint, Corbusier, Aalto, Oud and those in the Bauhaus and De Stijl schools promoted an assortment of anthropometrics, affordability, efficient use of space, mass production and housing for the general population (Imrie and Hall 2001, Marcus 1995). The Spanish architect Gaudi built properties with flexible components such as sliding room partitions to enable greater functionality within dwellings – his Casa Mila in Barcelona is a notable example. These movements never created a groundswell of adoption in architectural practice. Nor was architectural practice in most of the 20th century known for attention to lifespan issues and the 'non-average'. This was to be imposed on the field increasingly, beginning in the 1960s with the rise of the disability movement in the US and UK. The Joseph Rowntree Foundation is amongst the leaders in the UK promoting the building and designing of lifetime homes (Barnes and Mercer 2001).

Early in the 20th century, the field of industrial design developed in tandem with the fields of ergonomics and human factors. One can trace the more effective response of the industrial design field to usability issues and considerations than was the case with architecture. The accessibility field in the US and the UK has been part of the civil rights movement for people with disabilities that began after World War II, and was related to the larger worldwide human rights movement principally identified with the United Nations. The US disability activities paralleled other similar civil rights movements by disenfranchised groups in the US at that time, for example women, African Americans and Native Americans (Bickenbach 2001).

Since the 1960s, the disability community in the US has vigorously advocated for the creation of civil rights legislation and building regulations that provided accessibility features, e.g. kerb cuts, stepless entrances and lever door hardware. The initial major push for accessible building design came after the publication of the American National Standards Institute's (ANSI) 117.1 standard in 1961 (Salmen 2001), the first US accessibility design standard. In the UK the concept of wheelchair-standard housing only emerged in the 1970s following the introduction of The Chronically Sick and Disabled Persons Act 1970 Section 3, which placed a duty on local government bodies to consider the housing needs of physically disabled individuals. Other UK legislation and guidance that helped address accessibility issues, and which will be discussed in greater detail in Chapter 9, includes the following.

## Legislation directly regulating disability access standards in housing

▪ Building Regulations Part M – Public Buildings (1987)
▪ Building Regulations Approved Part M – Dwellings (1999) and amended (2000 and 2003) (OPDM 2006)

## Legislation with secondary influence on housing

▪ The NHS and Community Care Act 1990
▪ The Manual Handling Operations Regulations 1992
▪ The Carers (Recognition and Services) Act 1995
▪ The Disability Discrimination Acts 1995, 2004
▪ Housing Grants Construction and Regeneration Grants 1996, Part I
▪ Human Rights Act 1998 (Carroll *et al.* 1999, Chapman 1999)

## Design guides

▪ Joseph Rowntree Foundation – *Costing Lifetime Homes* (Sangster 1997)
▪ Social Services departments and Housing Authority collaboration guides
▪ Selwyn Goldsmith – *Designing for the Disabled* 1976

There was a general consensus amongst involved groups, including disability activists, that access and usability were limited and additionally that there was wide variation amongst guides; the need to develop a robust evidence base began to emerge.

In 2001 the British Standards Institute (BSI) published BS: 8300 *Design of buildings and their approaches to meet the needs of disabled people*, underpinned by a substantial ergonomic study of the spatial needs of 91 wheelchair users. This study is considered to contain the best ergonomic data currently available although the needs of individuals with sensory impairment and individuals with mental health and emotional impairments are less well dealt with.

Over the course of this roughly 25-year timespan the concept of universal design arose. The success of the accessibility work in the intervening years had made great progress by appearing in some governmental/federal and state policies with respect to programmes and services, architecture, transportation, public rights of way, public spaces and, to a lesser extent, housing. Although not uniformly nor consistently applied, by the mid-1980s accessible design was becoming more of a reality for the design and construction industry across the globe.

Although great gains were achieved for disabled people through the accessibility provisions some key flaws prevented it from becoming the necessary solution. Later analysis by Lusher and Mace (1989) showed that the standards '. . . have been developed by an approach of modifying the norm through the use of a few specially designed features and products to accommodate the "few" who vary from the norm' (p.754). The authors point out that this approach led to an 'after-the-fact' implementation of access features (even in new construction) which resulted in facilities which have their own 'functional limitations' and aesthetic problems. Other challenges were also noted. 'As architects began to wrestle with the implementation of standards, it became apparent that segregated accessible features were "special", more expensive, and usually ugly' (ibid.).

American and European commentators offer important insights into the goals and beneficiaries commonly associated with universal design. The European Commission notes, 'In most respects, the integration of older people and people with disabilities *into society* will only come about as a result of designing mainstream products and services to be accessible by as broad a range of users as possible' (Story *et al.* 1998, p.11). Story *et al.* assert that universal design should '. . . integrate people with disabilities into the mainstream' and that it will '. . . reduce the physical and attitudinal barriers between people with and without disabilities'.

The global social inclusion initiatives gathering momentum within the UK and across Europe echo these views – that true inclusion can be best achieved by mainstream integration, with two notable exceptions. Deaf people require inclusion and not assimilation and those with cognitive limitations require supervision and protective environments – mainstream provision for these groups may not be wholly appropriate. These concerns are discussed in Chapters 3 and 8 respectively (Barnes and Mercer 2001, Calkins *et al.* 2001). That will mean integration with the broad environment and making adjustments for the needs of those who use the environment differently. Universal design will yield advantages for everyone but will be of particular importance to people with disabilities (Danford and Steinfeld 2006, Ministry of the Environment Norway 1999). The disability movement is properly credited with creating the context from which universal design could materialise in the 20th century. The ageing phenomenon seems to be a prime driving force for universal design in the 21st century (Barnes and Mercer 2001).

## The principles of universal design (Center for Universal Design 1997)

The seven principles are presented here and each case is illustrated by an example.

Please note that although more than one principle may apply in each example, only one principle will be identified. Readers are encouraged to identify other principles and/or the guidelines within the examples themselves as an applied exercise.

### Principle one: equitable use

The design is useful and marketable to any group of users (Fig. 6.1).

### Guidelines

**1a.** Provide the same means of use for all users: identical whenever possible; equivalent when not.
**1b.** Avoid segregating or stigmatising any users.
**1c.** Provisions for privacy, security and safety should be equally available to all users.

### Principle two: flexibility in use

The design accommodates a wide range of individual preferences and abilities (Fig. 6.2).

### Guidelines

**2a.** Provide choice in methods of use.
**2b.** Accommodate right- or left-handed access and use.
**2c.** Facilitate the user's accuracy and precision.
**2d.** Provide adaptability to the user's pace.

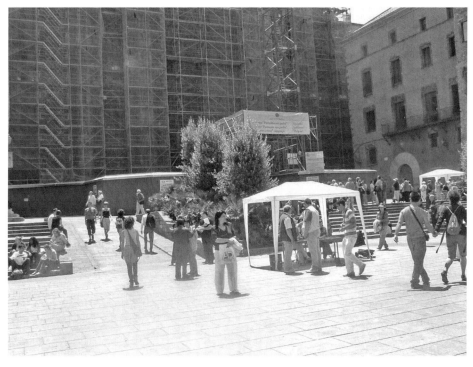

**Figure 6.1** Principle 1 Equitable Use. Barcelona cathedral, Spain. Ramped and stepped entrance promote equity in use.

### Principle three: simple and intuitive use

Use of the design is easy to understand, regardless of the user's experience, knowledge, language skills or current concentration level (Fig. 6.3).

### Guidelines

**3a.** Eliminate unnecessary complexity.
**3b.** Be consistent with user expectations and intuition.
**3c.** Accommodate a wide range of literacy and language skills.
**3d.** Arrange information consistent with its importance.
**3e.** Provide effective prompting for sequential actions.
**3f.** Provide timely feedback during and after task completion.

### Principle four: perceptible information

The design communicates necessary information effectively to the user, regardless of ambient conditions or the user's sensory abilities (Fig. 6.4).

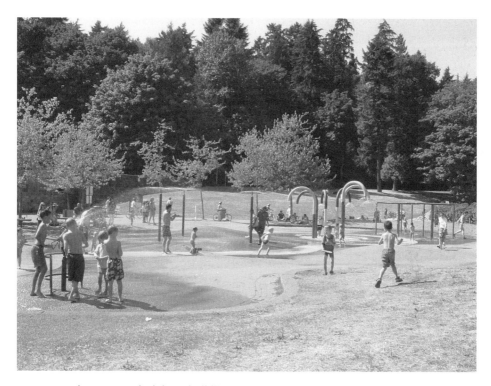

**Figure 6.2** Principle 2 Flexibility in Use. Stanley Park, Canada.

## Guidelines

**4a.** Use different modes (pictorial, verbal, tactile) for presentation of essential information.

**4b.** Provide adequate contrast between essential information and its surroundings.

**4c.** Maximize 'legibility' of essential information in all sensory modalities.

**4d.** Differentiate elements in ways that can be described (i.e. make it easy to give instructions or directions).

**4e.** Provide compatibility with a variety of techniques or devices used by people with sensory limitations.

### Principle five: tolerance for error

The design minimizes hazards and the adverse consequences of accidental or unintended actions (Fig. 6.5).

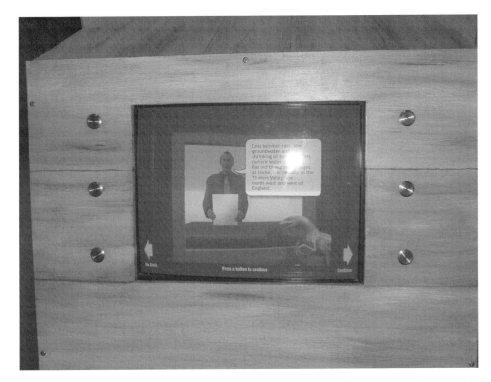

**Figure 6.3** Principle 3 Simple and Intuitive Use. Wetlands Centre, London, UK. This interactive information unit provides both visual and auditory information. The silver buttons along either side of the screen allow the user to navigate through the programme. There are no incorrect moves as each time the button is operated some interesting information about 'wetlands' is given.

### Guidelines

**5a.** Arrange elements to minimize hazards and errors: most used elements, most accessible; hazardous elements eliminated, isolated or shielded.

**5b.** Provide warnings of hazards and errors.

**5c.** Provide fail-safe features.

**5d.** Discourage unconscious action in tasks that require vigilance.

### Principle six: low physical effort

The design can be used efficiently and comfortably and with a minimum of fatigue (Fig. 6.6).

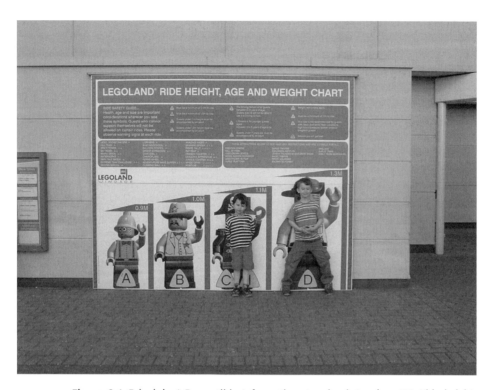

**Figure 6.4** Principle 4 Perceptible Information. Legoland, London, UK. Ride height, age and weight chart. Although the chart contains very important information this is easily conveyed to young children who have no difficulty in identifying which rides they will be able to take.

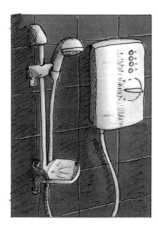

**Figure 6.5** Principle 5 Tolerance for Error. Thermostatically controlled shower. Prevents the possibility of scalding.

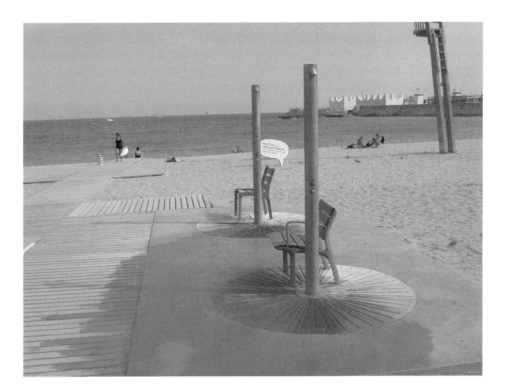

**Figure 6.6** Principle 6 Low Physical Effort. Wheelchair user's access to the beach in Barcelona, Spain. The boardwalk provides little resistance to propulsion.

### Guidelines

**6a.** Allow user to maintain a neutral body position.
**6b.** Use reasonable operating forces.
**6c.** Minimize repetitive actions.
**6d.** Minimize sustained physical effort.

### Principle seven: size and space for approach and use

Appropriate size and space are provided for approach, reach, manipulation and use regardless of user's body size, posture or mobility (Fig. 6.7).

### Guidelines

**7a.** Provide a clear line of sight to important elements for any seated or standing user.
**7b.** Make reach to all components comfortable for any seated or standing user.

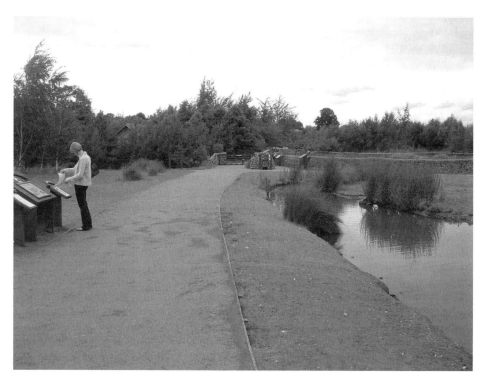

**Figure 6.7** Principle 7 Size and Space for Approach and Use. Wetlands Centre, London, UK. Wheelchair users' access to the information display is facilitated. Reach, manipulation and use are provided for a range of users.

**7c.** Accommodate variations in hand and grip size.
**7d.** Provide adequate space for the use of assistive devices or personal assistance.

At first reading, the principles themselves seem simple and almost commonplace. After all, most of us can readily identify how application of the principles even within our own lived experience will enable greater usability and inclusivity. However, the knowledge that underpins the principles is interdisciplinary, drawing from the fields of anatomy, physiology, psychology, ecology, occupational science, sociology, design and anthropology and doubtless many more, which is why these principles lend themselves to a broad application.

The principles are concerned with the 'top-down' perspective of how individuals interact with environments and artefacts in their endeavour of occupational performance. The greater the fit between the individual and the context of their occupations, the greater will be the satisfactory occupational performance outcomes. The principles propose a means, a system or an approach by which practitioners from a range of diverse backgrounds can organise knowledge from their

interdisciplinary perspectives through providing a structure for applying this knowledge in the service user's 'real-world' context.

Five key areas underpin the goal of inclusivity within UD.

1. Social equity
2. Ensuring a wide range of anthropometric fit
3. Reducing energy expenditure
4. Clarifying the environment
5. Using the systems approach

### Ergonomics, human factors and social equity

The final four of these principles come from the field of ergonomics:
the first two from the branch called anthropometrics and the second
two from the branch known as cognitive ergonomics (or human factors
in the US). The inclusion and integration of everyone in family, work
and community life are major goals of universal design. The ergonomics and human factors elements in principles 2–7 will drive a number
of decisions that will help achieve those goals. However, the primary
social equity instrument among the universal design principles is
found in Principle 1: Equitable Use. The design is useful and marketable to people with diverse abilities. In fact, without Principle 1 being
represented in combination with other principles (and specifically
Guideline 1d: Make the design appealing to all users) a universal result
is difficult to accomplish. This is the key component that drives inclusion. The emphasis on design integration and mainstreaming of features found in Principle 1 helps promote universal design in common
usage and common acceptance (Center for Universal Design 1997,
Mace *et al.* 1991).

### Misunderstandings about the meaning of universal design

Common myths include the following.

▪ That universal design is really 'just accessibility dressed up to look
good'. If this were true, a new paint job might suffice.
▪ That universal design is just *fully accessible* design but with the addition of characteristics that make it usable by other people too. Well-
engineered functionality is crucial to a universal outcome but will
always fall short if the design is not integrated or mainstreamed.
Often misused in this regard is the term 'universal access'.
▪ That universal design is an umbrella term that now covers all things
accessible and assistive. This lacks recognition of the broad beneficiary groups, the integrated and mainstreamed aspects of universal

design, and the differences between accessibility, assistive technology and universal design.
▪ A related idea is that universal design is the current term for accessible design. It is 'what we are calling it now'. This suggests the notion that universal design is merely the politically correct term that one must be careful to use in polite company (Danford and Steinfeld 2006, Mace *et al.* 1991).

Universal design and accessibility have continued to develop in a parallel manner. The philosophical bases for the accessibility movement and universal design are quite similar: inclusion, full participation and social equity. However, universal design extends beyond the confines of accessibility to include all persons and creates that inclusion by promoting integrated and mainstreamed products, environmental features and services.

## Beneficiaries of universal design

Over the last several years there has been a growing interest in universal design as an alternative to accessible design. Why has this occurred? In the highly developed countries there are several reasons.

▪ An increase in the number of survivors of disability.
▪ Increasing lifespans.
▪ Increasing purchasing power among the population with disabilities.
▪ Development of a 'grey market' with money to spend.
▪ Recognition of the inadequacies of assistive technologies.
▪ Products and environments that were not designed with old people in mind.

The world's altered demographics have strengthened the relevance of accessible and universal design. The ageing of many societies and the increased numbers of people with disabilities create a larger number of people who are obvious, immediate and significant beneficiaries of a more supportive environment. Often cited as the reason for considering a universal design approach in recent years, the changing demographics instead offer a reason for focusing on improved usability, safety and inclusion. Motives to include universal design features have been present for many years, as surely all human societies have included people with a wide range of human performance characteristics: tall, short, strong, weak, good and impaired hearing and vision, etc. The changing demographics provide an urgency to adapt design approaches and standards and to adopt universal design as policy and practice to catch up to the reality of the evolving international population (Mace *et al.* 1991).

As outlined earlier, the success of the accessibility movement in the US has created certain unintended challenges for universal design. The clear societal imperative to end discrimination against people with disabilities leaves a concept that is not particularly useful for the design process. The term 'the disabled' suggests a homogeneous group that has broadly similar needs, the uniqueness of each individual is hidden by the term and consequently the focus on individual needs is limited. The term 'disability' does not describe the individual or the group in a meaningful way. It groups all those to whom the term is applied (even if subdivided) into broad categories of impairment that lose specificity. It is therefore not helpful to say that something is 'accessible to people with disabilities' since each may have widely differing needs; for example, a ramped access will not particularly benefit a profoundly prelingually Deaf individual although clear textual and iconic signage might.

We know that people with disabilities have a vast range of abilities and impairments. A more useful way to consider the users of design is to understand the reality that we all exist along a continuum of human performance and other characteristics. We all vary widely in height, strength, visual ability, hearing acuity, mobility, balance, etc. An ergonomic approach is one technique that will help with implementation of the principles. Each person's characteristics can vary widely from each other and over time; someone who has a strong torso may have vision that requires the use of assistive technology to see adequately, e.g. eyeglasses. Someone who uses a wheelchair to move from place to place may have acute hearing, and so on. In spite of the frequent associations with accessible design and consequently with the misunderstanding that universal design is solely about design for people with a disability, universal design gives a general focus on the needs of all users ('user needs design'). This is a key distinction of universal design when contrasted with accessibility and assistive technology.

The consideration of friends, family and colleagues greatly multiplies the impact of more or less supportive environments beyond individuals to the social groups in which we all exist. Not to be forgotten are those who we might term 'circumstantially disabled'. These are people who, in the course of everyday life, find themselves operating differently because of their activities. Carrying a briefcase, coffee or a child will force any of us to alter the way we interact with the environment.

## Application challenges

An unfortunate response to the challenge of more accessible environments is to gravitate toward one of two extremes. One path is to mistakenly attempt to make everything 'fully usable by everyone' by abandoning creative, interesting and challenging designs. The other path that is sometimes followed is an unfortunate refusal to meaningfully engage with the issue by assuming that nothing can be done and that implementing an accessibility or universal design scheme will ruin the integrity of an existing building or proposed design. For example, a challenge is posed in large or complex environments, where it is sometimes not possible for each element to be universal in all respects. The inclination to make all outdoor play spaces fully accessible to children and adults with serious mobility problems is probably misplaced.

It is important to be creative about making as much as accessible as possible, keeping in mind all users – parents, grandparents, other family members – within the constraints of a particular project. Where physical access is not always possible, alternative means should be employed to provide comparable meaningful experiences. So a playground or recreation area might be quite universal while not having every place or every experience fully usable by all.

In other cases, it may be feasible to solve a universal design challenge at a larger scale. For example, fixed seating or benches such as those found in parks are typically installed at an average height, pitch and seat depth. Because users need widely varied seat types to accommodate variations in height, leg length, balance and postural requirements, many people are poorly served by single-style seating. Many modern office chairs today offer options, choices, adjustments and flexibility to respond to these personal variations. One solution might be to offer different sitting opportunities in the same seating area, whether with benches or other sitting opportunities. Although fixed seats designed to address one person's needs may be uncomfortable for others to use, providing different dimensioned fixed height seats in an array of seating might accommodate a wider range of users and produce a universal result in aggregate.

Taking the second path, with minimal engagement, can produce cursory results. For instance, some believe that single-storey homes are the only option for universal housing, ignoring the many opportunities for travelling between floor levels that are possible in a universal multi-level home. This effect is also encountered in the realms of historic preservation and renovations where a presumption may exist that nothing can meaningfully be achieved. Figure 6.8 shows a wheelchair user on a rooftop! In less developed outdoor environments such as parks and wilderness areas, a related fear is that of nature being paved over. In each case, a thoughtful and creative approach can produce surprisingly effective results that balance several competing interests. Figures 6.2, 6.6 and 6.7 illustrate this point.

Still, we know that universal solutions aren't possible for all situations. Individuals with dementia are one such group yet even here, by

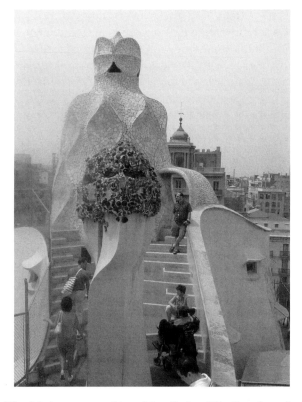

**Figure 6.8** Wheelchair user on roof top of Gaudi's Casa Mila, Barcelona, Spain. Keeping human diversity in mind, it is possible to provide good access almost anywhere!

combining the principles with dementia design, functional and aesthetic outcomes can be delivered, as discussed more fully in Chapter 8. More narrowly framed and targeted solutions (accessible and assistive technology) will always be required in cases where a particular feature does not meet an individual's needs. But the growth in the application of universal design will mean that those instances where additional, custom-made features are required will be fewer, less frequent, more limited and less costly (Duncan 2007). In such cases occupational therapists as specifiers should be able to apply the UD principles as far as possible to determine the usability of the equipment and communicate findings to the manufacturer.

## The boundaries of universal design

It must be acknowledged that the principles of universal design in no way comprise all criteria for good design, only universally usable design. Certainly, other factors are important, such as aesthetics, cost, safety, gender and cultural appropriateness, and these aspects should be taken into consideration as well.

The dominance of accessibility policy globally has created a number of specific means to balance accessibility and non-discrimination goals against other governmental and private interests. Because some goals of accessibility and universal design are shared, lessons may be transferable from one to another.

The most frequent trade-off encountered in universal design is that of affordability. This is the same concern heard over many years with respect to accessible and barrier-free features as well. Many suggest that an otherwise universally designed product or feature that is quite expensive may, in practice, not be considered universal because of its lack of affordability to many people. A case can be made that if universal features are only available at high cost, the limited access for many would be discriminatory. This is one reason why universal design proponents work to confirm and communicate the actual low cost of most universal features (particularly in housing). Those who are sceptical about accessible and universal design may cite high cost, especially when it is just for a 'few people's' advantage. The reality of broad beneficiary groups for universal design, discussed earlier, successfully counters this argument. It is becoming more difficult to assert that few are benefited by improvements to building usability (Steinfeld and Danford 2006).

Adapting existing buildings for accessibility can be expensive as they are virtually all renovation projects. There are running costs associated with poorly designed environments, these include staffing costs and associated risks to personnel. Some mechanisms for determining appropriate levels of added accessibility involve assessing the financial exposure of a particular entity in order to achieve a particular level of accessibility. Factors may include the size of an organisation, the costs of accessibility and the type of planned renovations, measuring the relative importance of an alteration compared to its financial impact on the entity that will pay for the capital improvements (Duncan 2007).

## Accessibility, assistive technology and adaptation

Universal design emerged from a world of special accommodations for people with performance characteristics that varied from what was regarded, at that time, as average. Whether accessibility features in buildings or assistive technology equipment at home or in workplaces, *special* and *different* were primary characteristics of many accommodations through the 1980s and beyond.

Universal design arose in part from the realisation that many of the 'specialty' design features characterised by accessible design turned out to improve life for others and have a much broader range of beneficiaries than was presumed. It also arose because the specialty features were often rendered in a way that limited the availability of their broader benefits. For example, special ramps leading to side entrances were much less appealing and useful than a level entrance that was easily traversed and obviously available to everyone, without forcing people to hunt for it or to navigate a longer, out-of-the-way route.

This idea of integrated design is represented in Principle 1: Equitable Use, and more precisely in Guideline 1d: Make the design appealing to all users (see Fig. 6.1). This fundamental social equity component was intended to 'raise all boats' in the rising tide of better, more useful and more supportive environments. There was never the expectation that a more universal world would eliminate all need for customisation of the environment to meet people's particular functional needs.

Even in a very universal world, all need for purpose-built, customised and specialised features and devices will not disappear. Rather, '. . . the idea is to improve the general environment in order to reduce the need for such settings and devices' (Steinfeld and Danford 2006, p.1) Universal design should become part of the standard process of achieving good design outcomes. 'Universal Design is a normative concept used as a goal in design of products, environments and communication systems' (Steinfeld and Danford 2006, p.2).

In considering the current definition of universal design, perhaps the term 'adaptation' itself should be removed or fully explained. Adaptation is unacceptable as a means of universal design if common understandings of the term are used: reconstruction, renovation or remodelling. This implies a good deal of effort and cost. However, designing for simple, low-effort alterations, similar to an idea of adjustment, is promoted as an acceptable route to universal design. This view underpins the naming of the environmental adjustment frame of reference introduced in Chapter 5. The distinction in name is important because a small-scale adjustment allows some design and user flexibility while maintaining user competency in interaction with the environment. It will also help achieve a mainstreamed appeal and affordability as expensive changes can be avoided.

## Principles revisited and future work

In spite of the progress that has been made in the field of universal design, it must be remembered that this field is still young. Accessibility itself has only been on the agenda for 50 years, seriously for only about 25 years. Universal design was only conceptualised about 20 years ago and the principles and guidelines are only marking their 10-year anniversary in 2007. Areas of potential remain relatively unexamined, much research is needed, the principles themselves might evolve, and practical implementation needs to be developed.

## *Areas of study*

Research is needed into:

- common reach ranges for standing and seated adults and children
- understanding and improving wayfinding methods in general, and ground surface types specifically, where great variations in theory and practice make consistency and true usability difficult
- identification of cognitive barriers and ways in which design can prevent undesired access and use for those with Alzheimer's disease and ways to address these through the principles of universal design. The fifth UD principle could address this issue partially but risk remains
- costs and benefits of universal housing, including health benefits
- the relationship between universal features, higher physical activity levels and increased community participation
- connections and collaborations between public health, planning and design professions, particularly with reference to social enterprise and social firm initiatives. Social enterprise and social firms have captured the interest of policy makers such as the WHO, the European Commission and many EU member states
- validated, practical environmental assessment tools
- best practice designs.

The fact that people increasingly live long lives is a positive sign of a prosperous and healthy society. It is an indicator of good public health, good health care, nutrition and occupational safety. The demographic trends in the developed world will not level off until the middle of the 21st century (Steinfeld and Danford 2006). Until then these nations will be in transition, moving towards a stable status of more equal age cohorts with only small diminutions at each level until the later years. During this worldwide transition, these societies will be coping with demographic changes in several key areas. The viability of pension and retirement programmes is being stressed, health-care costs are being stretched and caregiving systems are struggling to maintain services. All these systems will have to adapt to the changing population. By embracing universal design policies and planning, practitioners will be better able to handle those demands and ensure that quality of life values are included.

Norway is leading the world in its application of universal design. It has adopted the universal design concept and applied it more broadly and from higher levels of the federal government than is the case in the United States, the place of its birth, in making universal design and its philosophy an explicit part of broad national policy.

# References

Barnes C, Mercer G (2001) Disability culture: assimilation or inclusion? In: Albrecht GL, Seelman KD, Bury M (eds) (2001) *Handbook Of Disability Studies.* Sage Publications, California.

Bickenbach J (2001) Disability human rights, law, and policy. In: Albrecht GL, Seelman KD, Bury M (ed.) (2001) *Handbook Of Disability Studies.* Sage Publications, California.

British Standards Institute (BSI) (2001) *British Standard 8300: Design of Buildings and Their Approaches to Meet the Needs of Disabled People – Code of Practice.* British Standards Institute, Milton Keynes.

Calkins M, Sanford J, Proffitt M (2001) Design for dementia: challenges and lessons for universal design. In: Preiser W, Ostroff E (eds) *Universal Design Handbook.* McGraw-Hill, New York.

Cambridge Engineering Design Centre (CEDC) (2005) Cambridge University. Available at: www.eng.cam.ac.uk/inclusivedesign/index.php?section=introduction&page=employer-case2.

Carroll C, Cowans J, Darton D (1999) *Meeting Part M and Designing Lifetime Homes.* Joseph Rowntree Foundation, York.

Center for Universal Design (1997) *The Principles of Universal Design* (Version 2.0). North Carolina State University, Raleigh, North Carolina.

Chapman M (1999) *Guide to the Social Services 1999/2000,* 87th edn. Waterlow Press, London.

Disability Rights Commission (DRC) (2006) Available at: www.DRC.org (accessed July 2007).

Duncan R (2007) *Universal Design – Clarification and Development. A Report for the Ministry of the Environment.* Government of Norway, Oslo.

Fange A, Risser R, Iwarsson S (2007) Challenges in implementation of research methodology in community based occupational therapy: the Housing Enabler example. *Scandinavian Journal of Occupational Therapy* **14**, 54–62.

Goldsmith S (1976) *Designing for the Disabled,* 3rd edn. RIBA, London.

Imrie R, Hall P (2001) *Inclusive Design: designing and developing accessible environments.* Taylor and Francis, London, p.192.

Iwarsson S, Slaug B (2001) The Housing Enabler: An instrument for assessing and analysing accessibility problems in housing. Veten & Skapen HB & Slaug Data Management, Staffanstorp, Sweden.

Iwarsson S, Horstmann V, Slaug B (2007) Housing matters in very old age yet differently due to ADL dependence level differences. *Scandinavian Journal of Occupational Therapy* **14**, 3–15.

Kochtitzky C, Duncan R (2006) Universal design: community design, public health, and people with disabilities. In: M.M. General Editor, Editor. *Integrating Planning and Public Health: tools and strategies to create healthy places*. American Planning Association, National Association of County and City Health Officials, pp.51–63.

Lawton MP (1980) *Environment and Aging*. Brooks-Cole, Monterey, California.

Lawton MP, Nahemow L (1979) Social areas and the well being of tenants in housing for the elderly. *Multivariate Behavioral Research* **14**, 463–484.

Lusher R, Mace R (1989) Design for physical and mental disabilities. In: Wilkes JA, Packard RT (eds) *Encyclopedia of Architecture, Design, Engineering and Construction*. John Wiley, New York, pp.748–763.

Mace R (1985) Universal design: barrier free environments for everyone. *Designers West* **33(1)**, 147–152.

Mace R, Hardie G, Place J (1991) *Accessible Environments: towards universal design*. Center for Universal Design, North Carolina State University, Raleigh, North Carolina.

Marcus G (1995) *Functionalist Design*. Prestel-Verlag Publishing, Munich, p.168.

Ministry of the Environment (1999) *Government Circular MD-T-5/99, E part 1*. Ministry of the Environment, Accessibility and Planning, Oslo, Norway.

National Disability Authority (NDA) (2002) *Buildings for Everyone: inclusion, access and use*. National Disability Authority, Dublin, Ireland.

Office of the Deputy Prime Minister (ODPM) (2006) *Buildings Regulations Part M Amendment 2003*. RIBA Bookshop, London.

Ostroff E (2001) Universal design: the new paradigm. In: Preiser W, Ostroff E (eds) *Universal Design Handbook*. McGraw-Hill, New York.

Pheasant ST (1996) *Body Space: anthropometry, ergonomics and the design of work*, 3rd edn. Taylor and Francis, London.

Preiser W, Ostroff E (eds) (2001) *Universal Design Handbook*. McGraw-Hill, New York.

Reed K (1998) Theory and frames of reference. In: Neistadt E, Crepeau E (eds) *Willard and Spackman's Occupational Therapy*, 9th edn. Lippincott Williams and Wilkins, Philadelphia.

Salmen J (2001) US accessibility codes and standards: challenges for universal design. In: Preiser W, Ostroff E (eds) *Universal Design Handbook*. McGraw-Hill, New York.

Sangster K (1997) *Costing Lifetime Homes*. Joseph Rowntree Foundation, York.

Steinfeld E, Danford S (2006) *Universal Design and the ICF*. IDEA Center, University at Buffalo, New York, p.15.

Story MF (2001) Principles of universal design. In: Preiser W, Ostroff E (eds) *Universal Design Handbook*. McGraw-Hill, New York.

Story M, Mace R, Mueller J (1998) *The Universal Design File: designing for people of all ages and abilities*. Center for Universal Design, North Carolina State University, Raleigh, North Carolina.

Umbach S (2006) The changing scale of design. *Innovator* **Winter**, 4.

World Health Organization (WHO) (2002) *Towards a Common Language for Functioning, Disability and Health. The International Classification of Functioning, Disability and Health.* Available at: www.who.int/classification/icf.

Yerxa EJ, Clarke F, Frank G *et al.* (1989) An introduction to occupational science, a foundation for occupational therapy for the 21st century. *Occupational Therapy in Health Care* **6**, 1–17.

# 7: Knowledge from the field of ergonomics

In the previous chapter we saw how the principles of universal design provide an approach to guide the practitioner towards achieving more inclusive occupational performance outcomes for individuals. Yet the principles are broad and do not of themselves enable an application in practice. In order to implement the principles the practitioner is challenged to integrate the principles with knowledge from the field of ergonomics. This chapter will present an ergonomic theoretical framework to underpin the understanding of the relationship between ergonomics and occupational therapy, and to help the reader to understand and apply ergonomics to client-centred practice concepts (Mace *et al.* 1991).

By applying an ergonomic approach to designing inclusive environments practitioners can reasonably hope to achieve user-centred environments and products for service users. Phesant (1996, p.10) refers to five fundamental fallacies in design which should be avoided in practice if user-centred design is to be achieved.

1. The design is satisfactory for me – it will therefore be satisfactoiry for everybody else.
2. The design is satisfactory for the average person – it will therefore be satisfactory for everybody else.
3. The variability of human beings is so great that it cannot possibly be catered for in any design – but since people are wonderfully adaptable it doesn't matter anyway.
4. Ergonomics is expensive and since products are actually purchased on appearance and styling, ergonomic considerations may conveniently be ignored.
5. Ergonomics is an excellent idea. I always design things with ergonomics in mind – but I do it intuitively and rely on common sense so I don't need tables of data or empirical studies.

## What is ergonomics?

Ergonomics is defined by the International Ergonomics Association (IEA) as the application of scientific information concerning humans to the design of objects, systems and environment for human use. Ergonomics comes into everything which involves people. Work systems, sports and leisure, health and safety should all embody ergonomics principles if well designed (IEA 2007). It deals with the human–task demands that affect the individual during the course of those activities. These may be anthropometric, physiological, kinesiological, biomechanical, work design, workplace layout, cognitive and psychological demands (Kumar 2001). Pheasant (1996) suggests that work comprises many meanings; viewed narrowly as paid employment, the task is understood by its context rather than its content. When viewed more broadly as either paid employment or pursued as an interest or hobby, the context may have changed but the content remains the same and therefore the application of ergonomics is equally relevant and appropriate. 'It is the science of work; of the people who work and the ways in which it is done; the tools and equipment they use, the places they work in (including the home) and in the psychosocial aspects of the working environment' (Pheasant 1996, p. 4).

Trombly (1995) describes ergonomics as being concerned with the characteristics of people that need to be considered in arranging things that they use in order to determine the effective and safe interaction between both. Ergonomics, like the field of occupational therapy, is concerned with usability and environment and, like occupational therapy, also operates from a person–environment transaction perspective. Jacobs (1999) notes that occupational therapy arose from a belief that health is more than merely the absence of illness. Occupational science (Yerxa *et al.* 1989) is based on the inter-relationship between health and occupation (meaningful doing). The same could be said for ergonomics.

The ergonomic approach to design, according to Pheasant (1996), can be defined as the principle of user-centred design: any object, system or environment intended for human use should be based upon the physical and mental characteristics of its human users.

## History

The foundations of the science of ergonomics appear to have been laid within the context of the culture of ancient Greece. A good deal of evidence indicates that Hellenic civilisation in the 5th century BC used ergonomic principles in the design of their tools, jobs and workplaces (Ergonomics Society 2007).

The term 'ergonomics' (from the Greek words *ergon*, work, and *nomos*, natural laws) was first used by Wojciech Jastrzębowski in his 1857 article *An Outline of Ergonomics, or The Science of Work Based upon the Truths Drawn from the Science of Nature.* He believed that work, God's punishment to a wayward mankind, was also his consolation (Jacobs 1999). His views and those of occupational therapy are strikingly similar in that both believe in the benefits of work to humans. However, Jastrzębowski's theories were applied to the able-bodied population whereas occupational therapy applied its theories to those who were injured or ill (Jacobs 1999, Kumar 2001). Later in the 19th century, Frederick Winslow Taylor pioneered the 'scientific management' method, which proposed a way to find the optimum method for carrying out a given task. Frank and Lilian Gilbreth expanded Taylor's methods in the early 1900s to develop 'time and motion studies'. They aimed to improve efficiency by eliminating unnecessary steps and actions. This developed further during World War II, when scientists designed new advanced systems without fully considering the people who would be using them. It gradually became clear that systems and products would have to be designed to take account of many human and environmental factors if they are to be used safely and effectively. This awareness of people's requirements resulted in the discipline of ergonomics.

## Relevance of ergonomics to occupational therapists

Occupational therapists are interested in enabling individuals in achieving satisfactory occupational performance and we understand occupational performance to be a transaction between the task, person and their environment. Successful outcomes indicate good 'fit' between the components and this is also the interest of ergonomics; the salient difference relates to the populations with whom we each work.

Jacobs (1999) identifies five principal areas in which therapists can contribute to the practice of ergonomics:

▦ ergonomics for one (disabled individuals)
▦ ergonomics for special populations
▦ prevention of musculoskeletal injuries
▦ equipment design
▦ application of the disability discrimination legislation.

Jacobs (1999) further notes three major practice application arenas:

▦ workplace analysis aimed at prevention of work-related musculoskeletal trauma – MHOR 1992 ergonomic assessment requirement
▦ workplace tool design for disabled individuals

▨ research contributing to the development and use of databases – anthropometric data of disabled people or space/environment specification for disabled users.

Human factors, a discrete branch of ergonomics, are sets of human-specific physical, mental and behavioural properties which either may interact in a critical or dangerous manner with technological systems, human natural environment and human organisations, or they can be taken into consideration in the design of ergonomic human user-oriented equipment. Human factors tends to be the preferred term in the USA.

Often environmental demand is considered purely in terms of the physical environment yet the social environment also has a bearing on role and task performance. Beyond the physical environment, which also includes the people with whom we share our home, school or work place, the knowledge, skills, habits, expectations, values, attitudes and motivations of these people present conditions that support or impede task performance. Other influences that impact the social environment include cultural beliefs, norms, customs and practices (Neistadt and Crepeau 1998). These factors determine the overall tone and level of stimulation to which a person is exposed during task performance. For individuals with some mental health conditions or those with certain cognitive limitations, environments that place high demands on an individual's cognitive processing mechanisms or on one's affective and behavioural capacities can have a detrimental effect on task performance. Simply put, there is a transactional relationship and interdependence between the individual's capabilities, the task demands and the contextual environment (physical, social, cultural and psychological) that will positively or negatively impact occupational performance.

Pheasant (1996) suggests a methodology for using the ergonomic approach in practice, some of which will already be familiar to the occupational therapist.

During the 50 years of its history the science of ergonomics has gathered knowledge about human capacities and limitations and a repertoire of investigating methods for acquiring such knowledge and for practical problem solving. Two techniques in particular have proved very useful in these areas: task analysis and user trial. Task analysis is a formal or semi-formal attempt to define and state what the service user is actually going to do with the product/environment. This is stated in terms of the desired outcome of the task, the physical operations the user will perform, the information-processing requirements it entails, the applicable environmental constraints and so on. An effective task analysis will clarify the overall goals of the project, establish the criteria that need to be met, identify the likely areas of mismatch and so on – no doubt many readers will recognise elements of an occupational performance assessment in the foregoing.

A user trial is, as the name suggests, an experimental investigation in which a representative sample of the user population trial the end product/environment and determine its usability. Care should be taken to ensure that the trial conditions are as naturalistic as possible.

## The human–machine model

The simple human–machine model is of a person interacting with a machine in some kind of environment. The person and machine are both modelled as information-processing devices, each with inputs, central processing and outputs. This perspective can be seen to have congruence with the ecological conceptual practice models mentioned in Chapter 4 and can be particularly noted in the MoHO also based on a systems assumption. It proposes that the human system operates along similar lines to an information-processing mechanism. The inputs of a person are the senses (e.g. eyes, ears) and the outputs are effectors (e.g. hands, voice). The inputs of a machine are input control devices (e.g. keyboard, mouse) and the outputs are output display devices (e.g. screen, auditory alerts). In the human the central processing mechanism will be influenced by previous learned outcomes and an individual's cognitive capacity which will then produce outputs which in turn interact with the environment and lead to consequent inputs; the process is cyclical. The environment can be characterised physically (e.g. vibration, noise, zero gravity), cognitively (e.g. time pressure, uncertainty, risk) and/or organisationally (e.g. organisational structure, job design). Occupational therapists, by viewing individuals in this way, instinctively understand that by working with individuals to enable satisfactory occupational performance outcomes, intervention at the level of the input (broad environment) or the central processing mechanism (individual's capacity) can influence output (occupational performance).

In Chapter 5 the docility hypthesis was considered in detail and the associations with environmental press were noted with regard to the ageing population. Hall and Buckwalter's (1987) progressive lowered stress threshold (PLST) is a reworking of this with an application exclusively with cognitive impairment (Calkins *et al*. 2001). The point at which press exceeds the individual's capability is called the stress threshold. Hall and Buckwalter propose that where this threshold is crossed, dysfunctional behaviour occurs. Calkins *et al*. (2001) suggest that not enough has been written about why the environment causes these behaviours to occur and although it is helpful to have an understanding of models of memory and cognitive processing in relation to dementia, they note that this knowledge is not clearly identifiable in creating strategies for supportive environments.

## Product design

Even the simplest of products can be a challenge to use if poorly designed. Our ancestors didn't have this problem; they could simply make things to suit themselves. These days, the designers of products are often far removed from the end users, which makes it vital to adopt an ergonomic, user-centred approach to design, including studying people using equipment, talking to them and asking them to test objects. This is especially important with 'inclusive design' where everyday products are designed with older and disabled users in mind. Because there is very little measurement data available for certain populations, disabled groups being one notable example, it will very often fall to the occupational therapist to gather measurement data from the service users. This process will be discussed in detail under anthropometrics later in this chapter. Using learning from the field of universal design, practitioners can also make a judgement regarding the usability of assistive devices or other specialist equipment. Functionality of objects is important but reasons for non-use of equipment may also be linked to poor aesthetic value that may in turn cause the artefact to be viewed as stigmatising.

## Design to support cognitive impairment – healing and dementia design

Zeisel (2001) identified eight categories that appear to reflect specific brain abilities that have developed to help individuals cope with the environment and that need to be supported by the environment if people have impaired cognitive functioning in these areas. Table 7.1 identifies the specific areas of the brain, their capabilities and performance criteria for the environment and suggests design approaches known as 'healing design' to support performance.

Calkins *et al.* (2001) build on the seven principles of universal design to include additional guidelines that support cognition – a design concept known as dementia design. These are listed in Table 7.2. Both of these design concepts will be further discussed in Chapter 8.

**Table 7.1** Healing design performance criteria responsive to cognitive neuroscience. (After Ziesel 2001. Permission for use granted by MacGraw-Hill.)

| Brain location* | Brain capability | Design performance criteria | Possible design approaches |
|---|---|---|---|
| Parietal and occipital lobes | Ability to hold a cognitive map, ability to be in the present | The environment should provide the necessary information to help orientate the person to the physical setting rather than providing environmental demands (press) that require individuals to keep this information in their minds | Clarifying the environment, providing greater environmental legibility. Clear destinations, landmarks and pathways, all of these having a unique character that defines and distinguishes them |
| Anterior occipital lobe and hippocampus | Ability to hold onto the memory of objects and places | Environments that provide safety and security when a person is lost; clarity of surrounding environment; safety from external forces | Clear boundaries between home and public spaces; clarity of territory; ability to have privacy when needed |
| Frontal lobe | Sense of self | Personal environment that provides cues of one's own identity and autobiography | Moveable elements, furniture and decorations that evoke memories of a person's culture, personal history, family, achievements, etc. |
| Hippocampus and amygdala | Memory for places visited in the past; ability to retain moods, feelings and emotions | Spaces that evoke strong moods and emotions so that people feel – and thus know deeply where they have been | Varied spaces each evoking a different mood and emotion |
| Hippocampus | Ability to perceive and process new places; ability to retrieve long-term memories | Significant places that focus on hard-wired (long-term) memories such as food, warmth, social support, etc. | Environments that evoke strong hard-wired memories: fireplace, kitchen, garden view |
| Frontal lobe and motor cortex of the parietal lobe | Awareness of physical and other limitations and disabilities; sense of self-control and independence | Prosthetic environments that make adjustments for the loss of mobility or limb strength and that are safe | Environments with rails in hallways, accessible toilets, soft material on floors to cushion falls |
| Anterior and medial temporal lobe, and parietal lobes; sensory cortex | Receptive and expressive language centres; sense of smell, touch and hearing | Environmental cues in non-verbal form that use multiple sensory modalities at the same time | Environments in which sensory stimuli such as smells of food, sounds of music, comforting soft materials are arranged to augment written messages |
| Suprachiasmatic nuclei (SCN) | Sense of time and circadian rhythms; ability to sense nature, awareness of time passing and the seasons out of doors | Outdoor environment that provides contact with nature – natural cues to the passage of time | Gardens with clear pathways, planting areas, hard surfaces to walk on, benches to sit down on, shady areas, trees and plants |

* Note the information presented in this table is an oversimplification. Other areas of the brain may also influence behaviours and brain response.

**Table 7.2** Additional design guidelines that support cognitive functioning, known as dementia design. (After Calkins *et al.* 2001. Permission for use granted by MacGraw-Hill.)

| Universal design principle and guidelines | Additional guidelines | Strategies for implementation |
|---|---|---|
| **Equitable Use**<br>Provide the same means of use for all users: identical whenever possible; equivalent when not | Avoid confusion, promote continuity | Limit options. Use design elements, patterns and uses that are expected to be familiar to users |
| **Flexibility in Use**<br>Provide choice in methods of use. Accommodate right- or left-handed access and use. Facilitate the user's accuracy and precision | Avoid learning new concepts or means of use | Limit choices. Use design elements that are familiar to users |
| **Simple and Intuitive Use**<br>Eliminate unnecessary complexity. Be consistent with user expectations and intuition. Provide effective prompting for sequential actions and timely feedback | Innovation and intuition are often incompatible | Use expected imagery and standardised elements when possible. Use familiar and expected spatial continuum |
| **Perceptible Information**<br>Use redundant presentation; contrast between information and surroundings; maximise legibility | Avoid confusion. Enhance distinctiveness of important cues. Reinforce important information | Limit choices. Use non-standardised design elements. Use non-competing augmentative cues |
| **Tolerance for Error**<br>Arrange elements to minimise hazards and errors: most used elements, most accessible; hazardous elements eliminated, isolated or shielded.<br>Provide warnings of hazards and errors.<br>Discourage unconscious action in tasks that require vigilance | Error is unpredictable and can occur at any time | Accommodate selective access. Recognise that the most useable elements are often the most hazardous.<br>Recognise that error may result from intended as well as unintended actions |
| **Low Physical Effort**<br>Allow user to maintain a neutral body position. Use reasonable operating forces. Minimise repetitive actions. Minimise sustained physical effort | Minimise learning | Use familiar behaviour patterns when possible |
| **Size and Space for Approach and Use**<br>Appropriate size and space are provided for approach, reach, manipulation and use.<br>Provide a clear line of sight to important elements for any seated or standing user.<br>Accommodate variations in hand and grip size | Size should be appropriate for the type of use. Quality of space is as important as size | Reduce scale when necessary; provide private places for retreat |

## Size and shape

There will always be people with very particular needs so that customisation will be needed. Individuals with impairments fit into this category. In these situations it will fall to the therapists to determine the accurate size and shape of service users with respect to their person–environment fit. To this end the practitioner requires a method to implement intervention. This method is anthropometry.

## Anthropometrics

*Anthropos* means man and metrics is the branch of ergonomics which deals with measurements of the physical characteristics of human beings, particularly their sizes and shapes.

Anthropometry, the study of human dimensions, has many uses in design. Since its ascendancy in the period following World War II, engineering anthropometry has been used in the design of aircraft cockpits, automobile interiors, office and factory workstations, as well as homes and public buildings. What unites that list of domains is that they are all workspace dimensions – a place that the human must fit into – and this includes the artefacts (e.g. furniture) of that space. Anthropometry can also be used in the design of products which fit onto the wearer. Examples include general clothing, protective clothing, helmets of many types, gloves, masks, shoes, boots and so on. The design of products to fit onto the wearer is often characterised by sizing. That is, a bicycle helmet may be available in three sizes. Yet the design of workspaces, including all those domains listed above, is generally not sized; all human diversity is to be accommodated with only one size. There is one height for a doorway; there is one height for a counter in the kitchen. Some workspaces are adjustable, for example so-called ergonomic office seating or the six-way power seat found in many vehicles.

Only under very special circumstances is it possible to customise a product for a single user as this is not economically efficient. Some examples of this are haute couture, motor racing, astronautics and the rehabilitation of the severely disabled. It is with this latter group that occupational therapists work.

Anthropometrics aims to create products and environments which will accommodate as many people as possible with a variety of sizes, shapes and characteristics, also referred to as a target population. The aim in fitting the product to the user should be to achieve an acceptable dimensional match for the whole target population or the greatest possible number of the population. The variation in the size and shape of people also suggests that if you design to suit yourself, the product will only be suitable for people who are the same size and shape as you, and you might 'design out' everyone else!

Anthropometric measurements are compiled into tables and relate to different categories and population groups. These tables provide concrete and scientific information to support user-centred, functional design for the largest number of people. Anthropometry interfaces at the level of the person–environment–task transaction, to enable individual and work/task fit. Anthropometric tables are available for purchase although many are also available free of charge on the Internet (www.Ergonomics4Schools.com). There are very few tables available relating to physical impairment and those that are available are often unreliable (Bradtmiller 2000).

## Anthropometrics and populations with impairments

Ordinarily, in sampling for anthropometric surveys, a multidimensional matrix is drawn up to make sure that all critical sources of anthropometric variability are accounted for in the eventual sample. In the Army's most recent anthropometric survey, for example, the matrix included sex, race and age. This is because these three demographic parameters account for much of the anthropometric variability in a non-disabled population (IEA 2007). While the matrix approach is useful for the population of interest here, the same three parameters are not particularly effective. This is because the type of disability has much more to do with eventual body size and shape differences than it does with race, age and sex. These parameters are still important in defining a population of people with disabilities, so those parameters remain.

Dividing a wheelchair population into significant groups for sampling purposes is problematic. One approach is that suggested by Kumar (1997, 2001): when developing a sampling strategy for a pilot study, one would select the most frequent four or five conditions and group the rest into a category called 'Other'. For a full-scale survey, with a more complex sampling strategy, one would be able to use more specific categories and reduce the number in the 'Other' group. In most situations practitioners will be working with individuals and using individual measures only and so taking individual measures will be the focus of this chapter.

Appendix II lists anthropometric tables for a range of users in the general population. Disabled groups are not especially noted and are conspicuous by their absence so there is a pressing need for such data to be gathered and included within such tables.

In Chapter 8 a case study of a ward population is used to apply the universal design and dementia and healing design principles. Practitioners should be aware that most good design guides will have been compiled from anthropometric tables. It will also be possible to specify for environments through referring to scaled dimensions and relating these to reputable design guides (NDA 2002). When practitioners assess in group settings it will be possible to use accessible zones and the broad anthropometric range data, ensuring that both extremes are catered for (Jacobs 1999, Kumar 2001, Neistadt and Crepeau 1998, Pheasant 1996). In this case study it would be possible for the practitioner to take sample individual measurements of the 5th percentile (smallest) and the 95th percentile (tallest/largest) individuals to determine if there is good fit (some tables have broadened their population range to include all those between the 2.5 percentile and the 97.5 percentile).

Practitioners can use this knowledge in conjunction with application of the seven principles of universal design when designing environments for older people and individuals with impairments. A solid understanding of good design principles is essential for designing enabling environments for individuals with impairments and older persons. Disabling environments lead to exclusion and ill health. Using anthropometric measurements is one approach to designing optimal environments for service users; it is evidence based and user centred.

## Static and dynamic data

### Static (structural) anthropometry

Static or structural anthropometrics provides general, approximate figures that can be applied to a wide number of situations. Static anthropometrics measures the distance of bones between joint centres, including some soft tissue measurements in contour dimensions. It doesn't include clothing and therefore refers to a naked person.

Static anthropometric data is useful but you have to be very careful how you use it. The majority of the data refers to the measurement of a human in a static position, i.e. sitting in a chair or standing still. But when people move, those sizes probably don't reflect the actual size required. For example, when you walk your height 'increases' as you push off with your foot. There have been cases of doors being designed for the 90th percentile but people smaller than that were hitting their head as they moved through the door. It is the understanding of how people relate to their environment that is the ergonomics.

## Dynamic (functional) anthropometry

Dynamic or functional anthropometrics applies to specific situations and must be gathered as the situation arises. Distances are measured when the body is in motion or engaged in a physical activity. It includes reach (for example, arm plus extended torso), clearance (for example, two people going through a doorway) and volumetric data.

For example, forward reach may be measured by having a standing person stretching out their arm horizontally. This is a rather contrived pose and not one people usually adopt. Instead, when stretching to reach something, the shoulder might also be brought forward, and sometimes the body as well, to provide a longer reach. When reaching upwards, some might stand on tiptoe to reach the top shelf, etc.

This means that although the static figures can be used as a guide, it is also important to look at the situation which is being designed for. Occupational therapists should see their service users perform the required task and in this way both static and dynamic measurement can be recorded (Jacobs 1999, Kumar 2001, Neistadt and Crepeau 1998, Pheasant 1996).

## Distribution of measurements

Any population distribution (set of measurements) can be represented by three statistics: mean (the average), median (midpoint at which 50% >, 50% < than that point) and mode (most frequently occurring number).

### Normal distribution

In a normal distribution all three statistics, the mean, median and mode, are the same. Sixty-eight percent of values in a normal distribution are within one standard deviation (SD) of either side of the mean, 95% are within two SD and 99% are within three SD.

> Example: X = 60, SD = 4, 56–64 = 2/3 of everyone in the class
> + 2 SD, 52–68 = 95% of sample
> + 3 SD, 42–72 = pretty well covered the sample.

### Percentiles

Most data tables show the average and the two extremes of human size. These are the 50th, the 5th and the 95th percentiles, respectively. Male and female sizes are generally separate since there are big differences in the sizes of males and females. Occupational therapists inter-

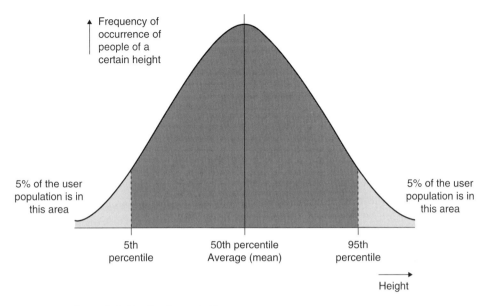

**Figure 7.1** Distribution or bell curve.

vene with individuals at the extremes of the general population range, usually at the 5th and 95th percentiles, i.e. with individuals whose capacities are at the extremes of human ability. When working with specialist populations, those at the extremes of this spectrum will be most disadvantaged by the environment.

Percentiles are shown in anthropometry tables and they express whether the measurement given relates to the 'average' person or someone who is above or below average in a certain dimension.

If you look at the heights of a group of adults, you'll probably notice that most of them look about the same height. A few may be noticeably taller and a few noticeably shorter. This 'same height' will be near the average (called the 'mean' in statistics) and is shown in anthropometry tables as the 50th percentile, often written as '50th %ile'. This means that it is the most likely height in a group of people. If we plotted a graph of the heights (or most other dimensions) of our group of people, it would look similar to Figure 7.1 which shows the typical population distribution, also known as a bell curve because of its shape! First, notice that the graph is symmetrical – so that 50% of people are of average height or taller, and 50% are of average height or smaller. The graph tails off to either end, because fewer people are extremely tall or very short. To the left of the average, there is a point known as the 5th percentile, because 5% of the people (or one person in 20) are shorter than this particular height. The same distance to the right is a point known as the 95th percentile, where only one person in 20 is taller than this height (Jacobs 1999, Kumar 2001, Pheasant 1996).

So, designers also need to know whether they are designing for all potential users or just the ones of above or below average dimensions. If a doorway is being designed by using the height, shoulder width, hip width, etc. of an average person, then half the people using the doorway would be taller than the average and half would be wider. Since the tallest people are not necessarily the widest, more than half the users would have to bend down or turn sideways to get through the doorway. Therefore, in this case the designer would need to use the dimensions of the widest and tallest people to ensure that everyone could walk through normally (Pheasant 1996).

Deciding whether to use the 5th, 50th or 95th percentile value depends on *what* you are designing and *who* you are designing it for. Usually, if the right percentile is selected, 95% of people will be able to use a design. For instance, if a designer was choosing a door height, then the dimension of people's height (often called 'stature' in anthropometry tables) and the 95th percentile value would be the critical dimensions to select; in other words, the designer would design for the taller people and all others below this height (below the 95th percentile) would be able to fit through the door anyway.

At the other end of the scale, if designing an aeroplane cockpit and reach was the critical dimension to make sure everyone could reach a particular control, then the 5th percentile arm length would be the critical dimension because the people with the shortest arms are those who are most challenging to design for. If they could reach the control, everyone else (with longer arms) would be able to. Similarly these criteria also apply within the field of occupational therapy when designing environments to support occupational performance.

Anthropometrics is concerned with the relationships between the dimensions of the user and the object, design or environment. For example, the relationship between the door height and the tallest man, the relationship of the chair to your optimum sitting height, the size of the mouse to the size of your hand. The relationships can be classified as relating to clearance, reach and posture.

- *Clearance* relates to the space that is available between the body, or body part, and the object; for example, space above doors (head room), under desks (for thighs, knees and legs), between the door and door handle. The clearance must be sufficient to accommodate a large-sized member of the population. In some top-of-the-range cars the roof is not sufficiently high to accommodate 95th percentile men.
- *Reach* should be based on the smallest member of the population to be designed for, so allowing the specification of the maximum dimen-

sion allowable. The top shelf in the supermarket needs to be reached by those with the shortest overhead reach.

■ *Posture*. Designing non-adjustable workspaces to ensure the best posture for a range of people is more difficult. For example, a kitchen worktop should be between 50 and 100 mm below the elbow height of the user when standing. The best height will be the one which fits the most people and causes the least amount of postural discomfort.

Many postural problems can be alleviated by adjustable furniture designed to accommodate the 5th–95th percentile range. Even so, users must be trained in how to adjust the furniture themselves and provided with good overall working conditions such as rest breaks, opportunities to change posture, etc. Although this may sound old-fashioned, currently much time is spent in stationary activities, especially in front of computers, leading to fatigue and muscle ache.

Designers have until recently tended to design between the 5th and 95th percentiles, which will accommodate 90% of the population. The reasons for this are pragmatic. Trying to accommodate all the population adds to the design constraints and becomes more costly, for less and less return. However, it is now more customary to design for 2.5–97.5 percentiles and to take more account of disabilities.

Before applying any anthropometric data to design decisions, the type of user who is going to work in the environment or use the product should be considered. For example, if designing sinks for primary schools, the designer should be considering the standing height of 6–11 year olds and not the teachers.

However, in many circumstances it is difficult to actually find and measure a large enough representative sample of the population you are designing for. For that reason, tables of data have been compiled and made available to practitioners and students (Pheasant 1996). See Appendix II.

Two of the most obvious factors that affect anthropometric measurements in the general population are sex and age. Women tend to be on the whole shorter and lighter; height increases until the late teenage years and then decreases again in old age (due to changes in the spine). Other factors include the fact that each generation is a bit taller than the one before, there are socio-economic and national differences, and certain occupational groups may be significantly different from the average population (for example, jockeys are shorter and lighter). Readers are referred to Stephen Pheasant's excellent work *Body Space: anthropometry, ergonomics and the design of work* (1996) for a more comprehensive account of the application of anthropometrics (Jacobs 1999, Kumar 2001, Neistadt and Crepeau 1998, Pheasant 1996).

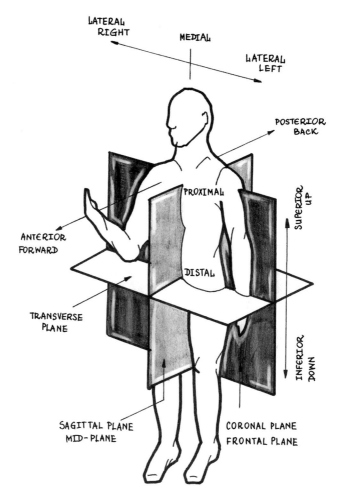

**Figure 7.2** Anatomical planes used in anthropometrics as points of reference for taking measurements. (Drawn by Kasia Halota.)

## Static anthropometric measurements – the measurement of human dimensions

Static anthropometry views the individual from one of two perspectives or planes: the sagittal or midplane, which divides the body into left and right views, and the coronal or frontal plane, which divides the body into front and back views (Fig. 7.2). Additionally, static anthropometry takes measurements from two standard postures – seated and standing.

- *Standard standing posture* (where this is possible). The individual stands erect, looking directly ahead and standing to full height and unsupported. Shoulders should be relaxed and arms should hang loosely at the side.

▪ *Standard sitting posture.* The individual sits erect on a horizontal flat surface, pulled up to full height and looking directly ahead. Shoulders should be relaxed and upper arms should hang freely by the sides with forearms in a horizontal 90° position. The thighs should be placed in a horizontal position and the lower legs should be vertical. The knees should be flexed at 90°. The feet should be at right angles to the floor and pointing forward. Readings are taken from a horizontal reference point, which is parallel to the transverse plane that is either the seat or the floor/ground, and a vertical reference point, a real or imaginary plane which touches the back of the uncompressed buttocks and the shoulder blades of the individual.

The following 24 human dimensions are considered to be the most common and have greatest relevance to occupational therapists in practice (Jacobs 1999). More extensive dimensions are available in Pheasant (1996). Figures 7.3 and 7.4 depict the standard standing and sitting measurement postures used in anthropometry.

1. Stature: the vertical distance from the floor to the crown of the head.
   *Application: defines vertical clearance in the standing workspace. Determines safe height for overhead obstructions, e.g. roof beams and light fittings. Determines bed length.*
2. Eye height: the vertical distance from the floor to the inner corner of the eye.
   *Application: centre of visual field, reach dimensions for sight lines and maximum height for visible obstructions Determines mirror and peep hole height.*
3. Shoulder height: the vertical distance from the floor to the acromion (bony tip of shoulder).
   *Application: the approximate centre of rotation of the upper limb, indicates ranges of comfortable reach. Reference indicator for fixtures, fittings and controls, etc.*
4. Elbow height: the vertical distance from the floor to the olecranon process of the elbow.
   *Application: indicates suitable range for worktop height.*
5. Hip height: the vertical distance from the floor to the greater trochanter (a bony prominence palpable at the upper end of the thigh bone).
   *Application: centre of rotation of the hip joint, functional length of the lower limb (shoes must be taken into account in dimensions and work area).*
6. Knuckle height: vertical distance from the floor to the third metacarpal (middle finger).

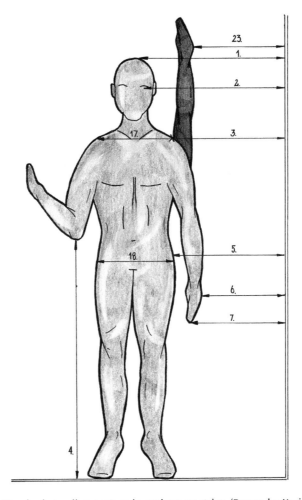

**Figure 7.3** Standard standing posture in anthropometrics. (Drawn by Kasia Halota.)

*Application: indicates the level for handgrips and rails for support. Approx. 100 mm above knuckle height is desirable.*

7. Fingertip height: the vertical distance from the floor to the tip of the middle finger.

   *Application: lowest optimal level for finger-operated controls.*

8. Sitting height: the vertical distance from the sitting surface to the crown of the head.

   *Application: the necessary clearance between seat and overhead obstacles.*

9. Sitting eye height: the vertical distance from the sitting surface to the inner corner of the eye.

   *Application: centre of visual field, reach dimensions for sight lines, and maximum height for visible obstructions.*

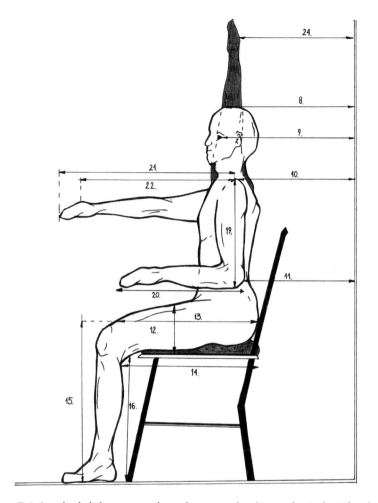

**Figure 7.4** Standard sitting posture in anthropometrics. (Drawn by Kasia Halota.)

**10.** Sitting shoulder height: the vertical distance from the sitting surface to the acromion.
*Application: approximate centre of rotation of the shoulder joint.*

**11.** Sitting elbow height: the vertical distance from the seat to the underside of the elbow.
*Application: heights of arm rests, key reference point in determining the heights of desk tops, key boards, etc.*

**12.** Thigh clearance: the vertical distance from seat surface to the top of the uncompressed soft tissue of the thigh at its thickest point, usually where it joins the abdomen.
*Application: clearance required between the underside of tables, desks, etc.*

13. Buttock–knee length: the horizontal distance from the back of the uncompressed buttock to the front of the kneecap.
*Application: clearance between seat back and obstacles in front of the knee.*

14. Buttock–popliteal length: the horizontal distance from the back of the uncompressed buttock to the popliteal angle, at the back of the knee, where the backs of the lower legs join the underside of the thigh.
*Application: reach dimension, defines optimal seat depth.*

15. Knee height: the vertical distance from the floor to the upper surface of the knee (patella) while in the standard sitting position.
*Application: clearance required between the underside of tables, etc.*

16. Popliteal height: the vertical distance from the floor to the popliteal angle at the underside of the knee where the tendon of the biceps femoris muscle inserts into the lower leg.
*Application: reach dimension, defines optimal seat height.*

17. Shoulder breadth: the horizontal distance across the shoulders measured between the acromia.
*Application: lateral separation of the centres of rotation of the upper limb.*

18. Hip breadth: the maximum horizontal distance across the hips in the sitting position.
*Application: clearance at seat level. Determines the seat width.*

19. Shoulder–elbow length: the distance from the acromion to the underside of the elbow in a standard sitting position.
*Application: determines upper arm support dimensions such as in seat back height and in rigid harness structures.*

20. Elbow–fingertip length: the distance from the back of the elbow to the tip of the middle finger in a standard sitting position.
*Application: forearm reach. Determines the normal working area.*

21. Upper limb length: the distance from the acromion to the fingertip with the elbow and wrist extended.
*Application: forearm reach. Determines the normal working area.*

22. Shoulder–grip length: the distance from the acromion to the centre of an object gripped in the hand, with the elbow and wrist extended and the shoulder flexed at 90°.
*Application: functional length of upper limb, used to determine range of comfortable reach.*

23. Standing vertical grip reach: the vertical distance from the ground to the centre of an object gripped in the hand with the shoulder flexed to a 180° angle (do not overstretch).
*Application: functional vertical reach in standing.*

24. Sitting vertical grip reach: the vertical distance from the seat to the centre of an object gripped in the hand with the shoulder flexed to a 180° angle (do not overstretch).
*Application: functional vertical reach in sitting.*

Figure 7.5 illustrates the broad-range anthropometric measurements from the 5th to the 95th percentile points.

## Anthropometric estimates for wheelchair users

For the most part, designers, architects and building planners have not deliberately avoided accommodating people with disabilities; they have been hampered by a lack of appropriate anthropometric data on which to craft a truly universal design.

A major nationwide anthropometric survey of individuals with disabilities should be conducted. Such a study would be designed to collect information including body sizes, reach capabilities, range of joint motion, strength and visual field data from several thousand children and adults, aged two and older, with a wide variety of disabilities. The resulting database would be widely useful to engineers, architects, designers and manufacturers of products that allow people with disabilities and the elderly to live independently (Bradtmiller 2000).

Accommodation and accessibility standards for individuals using mobility aids must take into account the wheelchair and its user as a single unit (Jacobs 1999). Figures 7.6 and 7.7 show the anthropometric postures for wheelchair users. All dimensions are with respect to the seat pan.

1. **Stature:** the first dimension is not applicable to wheelchair user dimensions as this dimension always refers to stature (the height of the individual when standing).
2. **Sitting stature/top of head height:** the vertical distance from the floor to the crown of the head.
   *Application: defines vertical clearance for the wheelchair user work space. The overall height space requirements will also be determined by the chair height including cushions.*
3. **Eye height:** the vertical distance from the floor to the inner corner of the eye.
   *Application: centre of visual field, reach dimensions for sight lines and maximum height for visible obstructions. Determines mirror and peep hole height.*
4. **Shoulder height:** the vertical distance from the floor to the acromion (bony tip of shoulder).
   *Application: the approximate centre of rotation of the upper limb, indicates ranges of comfortable reach. Reference indicator for fixtures, fittings and controls, etc.*
5. **Knuckle height:** vertical distance from the floor to the third metacarpal (middle finger).
   *Application: indicates the level for handgrips and rails for support. Approx. 100 mm above knuckle height is desirable.*

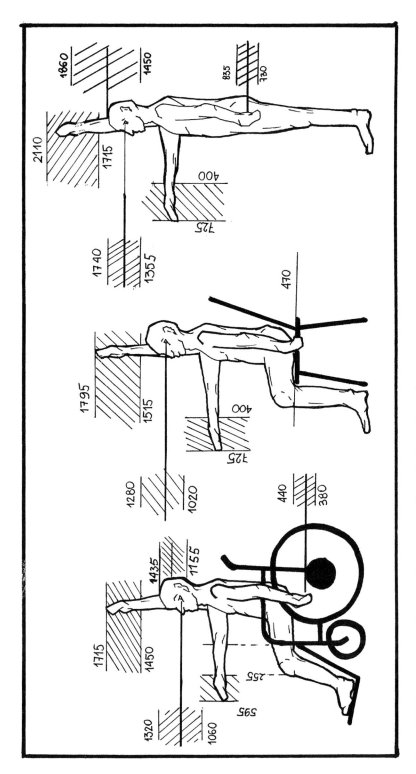

**Figure 7.5** Broad-range anthropometric measures. (Drawn by Kasia Halota.)

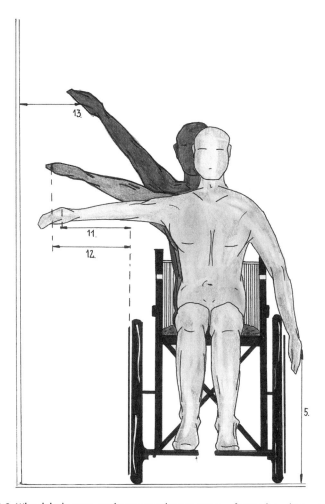

**Figure 7.6** Wheelchair user, anthropometric measures – front view. (Drawn by Kasia Halota.)

6. Thigh clearance: the vertical distance from seat surface to the top of the uncompressed soft tissue of the thigh at its thickest point, usually where it joins the abdomen.
   *Application: clearance required between the underside of tables, desks, etc.*
7. Toe height: the vertical distance from the ground to the top of the longest toe (phalanx) when supported in standard footplate position.
   *Application: clearance for foot.*
8. Shoulder–grip length/easy forward reach: the distance from the acromion to the centre of an object gripped in the hand, with the elbow and wrist extended and the shoulder flexed at 90°.

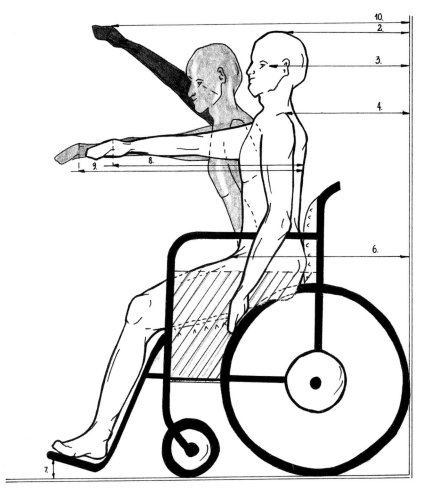

**Figure 7.7** Wheelchair user, anthropometric measures – side view. (Drawn by Kasia Halota.)

*Application: functional length of upper limb, used to determine range of comfortable reach.*

9. Maximum forward reach: the distance from the acromion to the centre of an object gripped in the hand, with the elbow and wrist extended, the shoulder flexed at 90° and the trunk flexed forward where it meets the pelvis.

*Application: functional length of upper limb, used to determine range of maximum reach.*

10. Floor to high forward reach: the vertical distance from the ground to the centre of an object gripped in the hand with the shoulder flexed to a 130° angle (do not overstretch) and the trunk flexed forward where it meets the pelvis.

*Application: functional forward reach in wheelchair.*

11. Easy side reach: the distance from the acromion to the centre of an object gripped in the hand, with the elbow and wrist extended and the shoulder abducted at 90°.
    *Application: functional length of upper limb, used to determine range of comfortable side/lateral reach.*
12. Maximum side reach: the distance from the acromion to the centre of an object gripped in the hand, with the elbow and wrist extended and the shoulder abducted at 90° and lateral flexion and rotation at the lumbar spinal region.
    *Application: functional length of upper limb, used to determine range of comfortable side/lateral reach.*
13. Floor to high side reach: the vertical distance from the ground to the centre of an object gripped in the hand with the shoulder abducted/side elevated to a 130° angle (do not overstretch) and lateral flexion at the trunk with rotation at the lumbar spinal region.
    *Application: functional length of upper limb, used to determine range of maximum side/lateral reach in wheelchair.*

### Limitations of static anthropometric estimates

Anthropometrics is not an exact science and in practice anthropometric criteria provide a guide rather than an absolute (Jacobs 1999). The human body is challenging to measure due to its form and consistency (rounded and soft) and when this fact is coupled with the difficulty of controlling posture (floppy or rigid), an accuracy of more than 5 mm is difficult to achieve (Jacobs 1999, Kumar 2001, Neistadt and Crepeau 1998, Pheasant 1996).

## References

Bradtmiller B (2000) Ergonomics: An Emerging Technology for Increasing Participation in Work and Daily Living. Paper presented at the RESNA Annual Conference and Research Symposium. RESNA, Arlington, Virginia. Available at: publications@resna.org

Calkins M, Sanford J, Proffitt M (2001) Design for dementia: challenges and lessons for universal design. In: Preiser W, Ostroff E (eds) *Universal Design Handbook*. McGraw-Hill, New York.

Ergonomics Society. Available at: www.ergonomics.org.uk/ (accessed July 2007).

Hall G, Buckwalter K (1987) Progressively lowered stress threshold: a conceptual model for care of adults with alzheimer's disease. *Archives of Psychiatric Nursing* **1**(6), 399–406.

International Ergonomics Association (IEA). Available at: www.internationalergon omicsassociation.com.

Jacobs K (1999) *Ergonomics for Therapists*, 2nd edn. Butterworth-Heineman, New York.

Kumar S (ed.) (1997) *Perspectives in Rehabilitation Ergonomics*. Taylor and Francis, Bristol, Pennsylvania.

Kumar S (2001) *Multidisciplinary Approach to Rehabilitation*. Butterworth-Heineman, New York.

Mace R, Hardie G, Place J (1991) *Accessible Environments: towards universal design*. Center for Universal Design, North Carolina State University, Raleigh, North Carolina.

National Disability Authority (NDA) (2002) *Buildings for Everyone: inclusion, access and use*. National Disability Authority, Dublin, Ireland.

Neistadt E, Crepeau E (eds) (1998) *Willard and Spackman's Occupational Therapy*, 9th edn. Lippincott Williams and Wilkins, Philadelphia.

Pheasant ST (1998) *Body Space: anthropometry, ergonomics and the design of work*, 3rd edn. Taylor and Francis, London.

Trombly C (1995) *Occupational Therapy for Physical Disability*, 4th edn. Williams and Wilkins, Baltimore, Maryland.

Zeisel J (2001) Universal design to support the brain and its development. In: Preiser W, Ostroff E (eds) *Universal Design Handbook*. McGraw-Hill, New York.

# 8: Applied examples

A practice example using ergonomics for special populations has been selected so that a broad range of impairments can be considered from the universal design perspective. The population presented is older people with Alzheimer's disease, which will provide opportunties for the practitioner to explore how the principles of universal design attempt to meet the needs of this group with physical, cognitive and sensory impairment. Consideration of carers' manual handling needs will also be included. The functional limitations resulting in the mismatch between impairments and environmental demands can also be applied to practitioners' individual cases.

## Reason for environmental assessment

- To determine the level of accessibility and usability of the ward environment for older persons with Alzheimer's disease. The proposed user population was likely to be individuals with limitations of functional mobility, sensory (visual and auditory), cognitive (memory and executive skills) and perceptual processing. This report also considers how the ward environment will support those with continence difficulties and the other attendant conditions of old age.
- To determine the level of accessibility and usability of the ward environment from an ergonomic and manual handling perspective for carers and staff during routine work performance tasks.

## Location of assessment

The older persons unit is currently undergoing rebuilding and refurbishment so a site visit could not take place. However, 1 : 100 scaled drawings of the proposed new ward were available for review (see Fig. 8.1 for plan detail). Additionally, although rather late in the rebuild

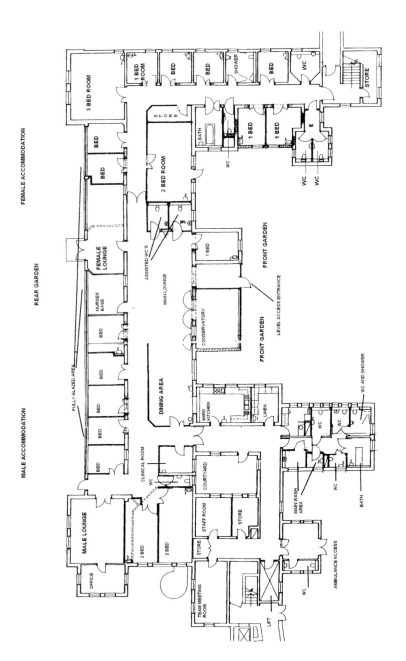

**Figure 8.1** Plan of the older persons unit.

SCALE 1:100

process, occupational therapists were invited to a ward planning meeting to advise on any environmental adjustments that needed to be considered for the proposed ward population.

The plan view of the older persons unit is similar to many wards in old institutional asylum settings. The dimensions are not included in the figure as the information would then be difficult to read but dimensions are referred to throughout the example.

**Ward** (type of accommodation, amenities)

Twenty-three bedded unit with separate male and female accommodation. The sleeping accommodation is a combination of single provision and two- (×3) and three-bedded (×1) provision. The predominant provision is for single-bedded (×14) occupancy. The single bedrooms are small (smallest at 2700 × 2700 mm) and will pose some mobility restrictions for some patients when all furniture and (as necessary) commodes are in place. The bedrooms are not en suite although 12 have hand basins provided.

Eight of the bedrooms across both male and female sections of the ward (identified from the plans/drawings only) appear to have large wall-to-wall windows. These rooms will offer excessive brightness and glare and will pose some difficulty for those with cataracts and other visual processing difficulties. Additionally, there will be reduced opportunity for personalising bedroom areas which may further impact on orientation and confusion with this population group.

There are separate male and female washing facilities. The male provision is predominantly located in a lobbied WC ×4/bath/shower block with two WCs located separately from each other and at some distance from the main male block. Circulation within the male WC block will be difficult for any patients using mobility equipment. In the event of a patient sustaining a fall in this area manual handling/transfer assistance could not be provided through use of a mobile hoist as there is insufficient turning circle space (minimum recommended is 1700 mm); this may pose a risk of cumulative manual handling injury to staff required to assist the fallen patient.

The female provision of seven WCs is located separately within the female section of the ward and is configured in two adjacent units of two. A further two (one having a level access shower) are located in close proximity and are separated by a bedroom (this is not ideal siting for a bedroom). The seventh is located adjacent to the bathroom. There is no female WC block as such, which may cause difficulty for some confused patients in locating the WC area.

Both baths are sited in peninsular style. Fixed ceiling track hoists should be provided to facilitate safe manual handling and afford patient dignity. Bathing/cleaning activity is predicted to be high given the likely incontinence and confusion of the patients (accidents are also predicted to be associated with not getting to the WC in time because of configuration). Consideration should also be given to the provision of over-bath or over-shower stretchers to facilitate staff in manual handling during patient hygiene tasks.

There is one kitchen in the ward and this serves as both ward and therapeutic/assessment kitchen. The detail of this area was not available at the time of the assessment. Recommendations on flexible kitchen design to accommodate a range of service users are provided later in the report.

It was unclear at the point of writing this report if the patients will access the day hospital sited approximately 500 m distant from the unit during their assessment stay at the older persons unit. If patients do visit the day hospital there will be additional difficulties in accessing this area since it is located some distance from the ward. Independent way finding would be difficult. Ideally, the day hospital and ward should be sited close to each other. However, the constraints of retro-fitting and refurbishment prevent this.

The ward has level access throughout and there is a garden to the front and rear, which could be developed as a sensory garden for the benefit of the patients. It is proposed that patients will have access to this area. Any stepped entrances to the ward should be ramped following the appropriate building regulations.

The ward provides a shared dining and lounge area in addition to two single-sex lounges. The female-only lounge leads directly onto the rear garden and any stepped entrance should be ramped.

## Client's performance capacity (mental state, physical, perceptual and sensory needs)

The proposed client group for this environment is older people over 75 years of age with mental health problems and/or dementia and deteriorating physical (including neurological) functioning. In such cases the environmental design and lay-out play a key role in facilitating or impeding performance and participation in the life of the unit.

The key areas of functional limitations may include some of the following.

■ Difficulty interpreting information
■ Diminished sight
■ Diminished hearing
■ Prevalence of poor balance

- In-coordination
- Limitations of stamina
- Difficulty in moving head
- Difficulty in reaching with arms
- Difficulty in handling and fingering
- Loss of upper extremity skills
- Difficulty bending, kneeling, walking, etc.
- Reliance on walking aids
- Reliance on wheelchair
- Difficulty sensing temperature (risk of burns during washing)
- Extremes of size and weight
- Difficulty in managing personal/intimate hygiene related to incontinence (Iwarsson and Isaacsson 1996)

## Potential impact of functional limitations on occupational performance imposed by the ward environment

The likely impact on occupational performance may include some of the following.

- Difficulty in way finding and remembering routes around the unit (due to cognitive deficit and some illogical circulation routes within the unit).
- Difficulty in following instructions (written and spoken).
- Difficulty in orientation to time, person and place and consequent self-imposed restriction of mobility due to fear of falls and/or fear of becoming lost on the unit.
- Difficulty with general mobility (including mobilising with mobility equipment) due to increased frailty and high-friction (thick carpet) and low-friction (linoleum) flooring within the unit. These surfaces are particularly hazardous in relation to wheelchair propulsion and mobile hoist manoeuvre and when mobilising with mobility aids (requiring increased effort on thick carpet and poor control on linoleum). The use of linoleum additionally increases the risk of falls due to liquid spills and generally does not wear well over time with heavy traffic (clients with mobility aids, wheelchairs and other wheeled equipment such as mobile hoists).
- Difficulty with manipulation of objects (dressing, feeding, using taps, operating switches and opening doors/cupboards/drawers, etc.).
- Prevalence of falls and related anxiety and/or further injury.
- Difficulty with transfers due to limitations of space and approach in bedroom and bathroom/WC and shower areas.
- Prevalence of soiled clothing and consequent risk of skin breakdown, infection and illness and loss of dignity.

- Prevalence of wandering due to confusion and/or diminished visual acuity. Environmental cueing can improve orientation and way finding by good use of colour contrasts throughout the environment.
- Prevalence of aggressive behaviour related to anxiety and agitation associated with mismatch between environmental demands and individual's functional capacities (Zeisel 2001).

## Summary of strengths and challenges

The new older persons ward provides some advantages to those admitted to this environment. These include:

- the provision of a garden to the front and rear of the unit
- level access environment throughout the unit
- separate male and female areas
- mixed gender areas
- a ward/assessment kitchen.

There are many challenges that should be addressed and rectified before the rebuild of the ward is complete. It is understood that there were limited resources available to complete this work and so compromises have been necessary. Some of the difficulties the environment poses to its potential client group include:

- small singe bedrooms that may not support safe transfers
- no en suite facilities – clients with continence difficulties may soil clothing
- lack of female WC block – may cause confusion in locating space
- proposed low-friction flooring (linoleum) may cause difficulty in mobilising and in using equipment. Medium-friction flooring may be the most appropriate option
- male WC area is restricted in space and approach, so safe transfers using mobility equipment may not be possible in this area. Many of the cubicle doors open out into the corridor area with consequent risk of injury to others
- the circulation within the ward could be potentially disorientating for service users unless colour contrasts and cueing are used to good effect
- presence of large areas of glass may cause glare, which may be further accentuated if high-sheen surfaces are used
- little possibility to meaningfully personalise rooms because of restricted space
- shared ward and assessment kitchen
- limited storage space for equipment within the ward
- garden area requires development as sensory garden.

## Applied universal and dementia design principles

The remainder of this chapter provides best practice guidance based on two design approaches.

■ The seven principles of universal design.
■ The five principles of dementia design.

The dementia design principles will be discussed later in the chapter following application of the universal design principles. The dominant universal design principles are noted in **bold** within the environmental features presented but many of the seven principles will apply to more than one setting simultaneously.

The information in the following section is drawn primarily from *Buildings for Everyone* (2001) published by the National Disability Authority, Ireland.

### *Access and circulation*

*Universal Design Principles: **Equitable Use**, Flexibility in Use, Simple and Intuitive Use, Perceptible Information, Tolerance for Error, **Low Physical Effort**, **Size and Space for Approach and Use**.*

Figure 8.2 shows the anthropometric data for space requirements for a range of users. It demonstrates the clear space required by people using different mobility aids. As will be seen later in the chapter, a path or corridor width of 1800 mm will allow a wheelchair user comfortably to pass another wheelchair user or someone using crutches.

#### Consequences for design and management

##### In the external environment

■ Avoid long travel distances and slopes. A distance or gradient which is easy for most ambulant people can be impossible for a person with a walking frame or using a wheelchair.
■ Some surface finishes, such as loose pebbles or badly maintained footpaths, present hazards and can make wheelchair use impossible.
■ On the footpath, even a small kerb can be hazardous or impossible to climb or descend.

##### Inside buildings

■ Long horizontal distances can be arduous or hazardous to accomplish.
■ Opening and closing doors is often difficult.

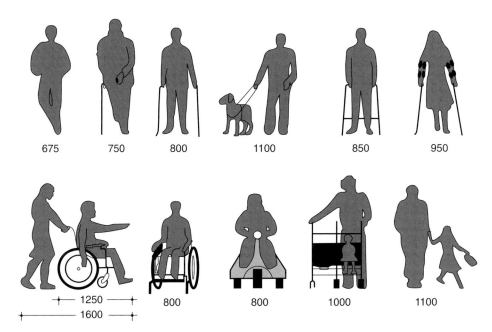

**Figure 8.2** Space requirements. (Reproduced with kind permission from *Buildings for Everyone*, 2002, National Disability Authority, Ireland.)

- A pair of narrow doors can be particularly disabling for people carrying shopping, accompanied by children or using a wheelchair.
- Space requirements for wheelchair users are greater than for ambulant people. A wheelchair is a rigid item which cannot, for example, squeeze through confined spaces. Be aware of this, especially in traditionally confined areas such as small lobbies and WC cubicles.
- Steps and staircases can be difficult or impossible to negotiate.
- Some floor finishes, particularly deep pile carpets, can make wheelchair use impossible.
- Other floor finishes – slippery tiles or polished linoleum, timber or synthetic flooring – can present a hazard to ambulant people.

Figure 8.3 shows the minimum space requirements (mm) needed to facilitate safe circulation along corridors by a range of users. Corridors for general public access should be at least 1800 mm wide to allow two wheelchair users to pass without difficulty. Other corridors must be at least 1200 mm wide. A wheelchair user should never be forced to reverse, as it can be a very difficult manoeuvre.

### Corridors

- Corridors to which the public has access should be at least 1800 mm wide.

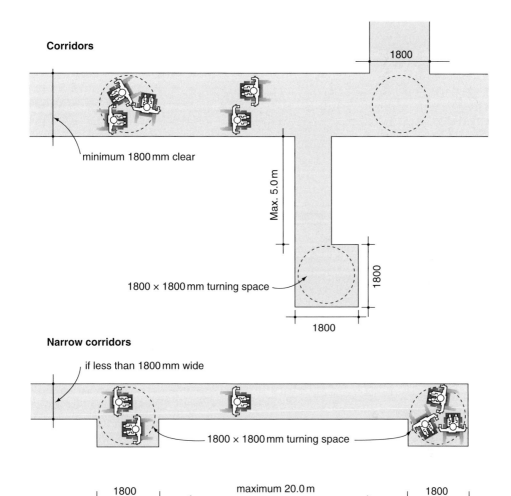

**Figure 8.3** The minimum space requirements (mm) needed to facilitate safe circulation along corridors by a range of users. (Reproduced with kind permission from *Buildings for Everyone*, 2002, National Disability Authority, Ireland.)

- Other corridors to be minimum 1200 mm wide, with turning spaces.
- Provide handrails on all corridors, and seating in those over 20 m long.
- Do not allow objects to obtrude more than 100 mm into width of corridor.

Figures 8.4 and 8.5 show stairs and handrail specifications.

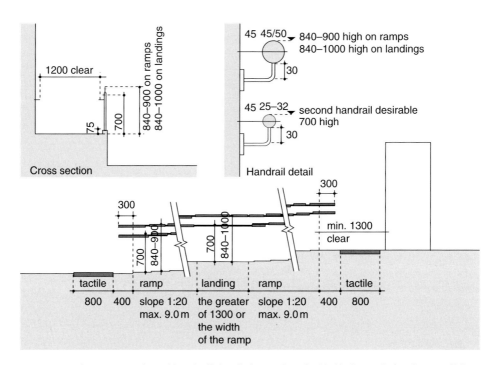

**Figure 8.4** Stair and handrail detail. (Reproduced with kind permission from *Buildings for Everyone*, 2002, National Disability Authority, Ireland.)

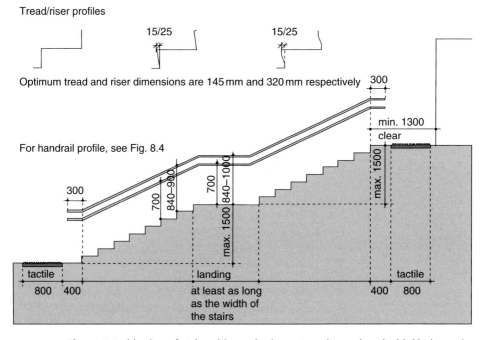

**Figure 8.5** Side view of stairs with emphasis on steps. (Reproduced with kind permission from *Buildings for Everyone*, 2002, National Disability Authority, Ireland.)

## *Doors*

*Universal Design Principles: **Equitable Use**, Flexibility in Use, Simple and Intuitive Use, Perceptible Information, Tolerance for Error, **Low Physical Effort, Size and Space for Approach and Use**.*

### Door type selection

▪ External doors should be readily identifiable, easy to operate and adequate in size.
▪ Provide glazed panels 900–1500 mm over floor/ground in corridor/external doors.

### Doorway planning

▪ Do not install doors unless necessary for functional or safety reasons.
▪ Provide clear space to door approach where in deep recess.
▪ Provide door clearance of 850 mm where corridors are 1200 mm wide.
▪ Provide 500 mm, minimum 300 mm, space at leading edge of door for wheelchair user to open door while clear of door swing. Figure 8.6 shows clear space at leading edge of door.
▪ Hang doors so as to open against an adjacent wall. Figure 8.7 shows door swing and closer detail.
▪ Do not allow doors to open onto ramps or circulation areas.
▪ Provide alternative unobstructed access beside turnstiles.
▪ Do not use revolving doors.

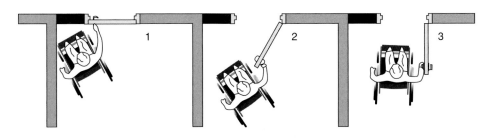

▮ 500 mm clear

**Figure 8.6** 500 mm clearance to leading edge of door on red side. (Reproduced with kind permission from *Buildings for Everyone*, 2002, National Disability Authority, Ireland.)

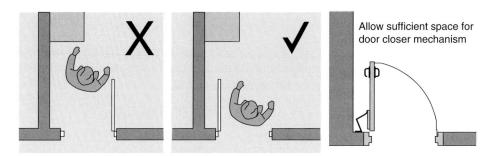

**Figure 8.7** Door swing and hang. (Reproduced with kind permission from *Buildings for Everyone*, 2002, National Disability Authority, Ireland.)

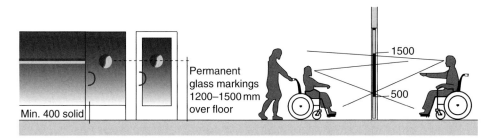

**Figure 8.8** Glazed door with sight lines identified. (Reproduced with kind permission from *Buildings for Everyone*, 2002, National Disability Authority, Ireland.)

## Dimensioning

- Minimum clear opening width to be 800 mm.
- In double door sets, at least the leading leaf to be 800 mm, but preferably both leaves.

### Glazed doors (Fig. 8.8)

- Mark glazing in doors and screens permanently at 1200–1500 mm over floor level.

### Powered doors

- Provide powered doors where practicable, particularly where manually operated doors would be heavy or difficult to open.
- Use presence sensors to detect movement in path of door travel.
- Provide button controls in accessible location.
- Provide adequate space to accommodate door-closing devices to ensure 800 mm opening.

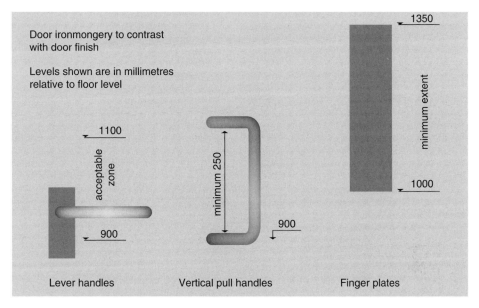

**Figure 8.9** Door furniture. (Reproduced with kind permission from *Buildings for Everyone*, 2002, National Disability Authority, Ireland.)

## Door furniture (Fig. 8.9)

- Hardware which is to be operated should contrast in colour with door leaf.
- Site door controls at height for both seated and standing users.
- Locate letter boxes 900 mm above ground level.
- Keyholes should be located above the handle, rather than below, to facilitate people with impaired vision.
- If a door closer is necessary, ensure it is delayed-action or slow-action type with gentle closing force (12N).
- Use cranked hinges where necessary to achieve requisite opening widths. Kick plates, where provided, should be minimum 400 mm high.
- Site and dimension pull handles to allow knuckles to clear adjacent frames or leaves.

## *Kitchen – ward and therapeutic (Figs 8.10 and 8.11)*

*Universal Design Principles:* **Equitable Use**, **Flexibility in Use**, *Simple and Intuitive Use*, **Perceptible Information**, *Tolerance for Error, Low Physical Effort*, **Size and Space for Approach and Use**.

- Plan flexibly, to allow for different users: sufficient space, simple layouts.

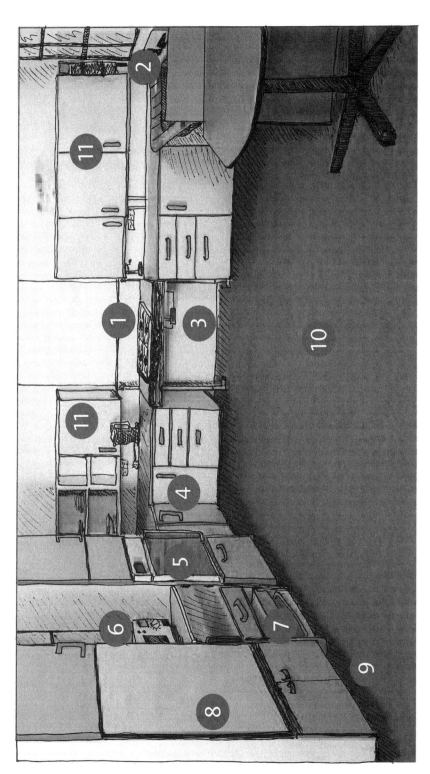

**Figure 8.10** Wheelchair-accessible kitchen. (Reproduced with kind permission from *Buildings for Everyone*, 2002, National Disability Authority, Ireland.)

1 Wall-mounted, height-adjustable hob
2 Wall-mounted, height-adjustable sink unit with lever taps and swan neck
3 Knee space under hob
4 Carousel unit to facilitate easy access
5 Oven with side-hung door at accessible level
6 Microwave oven with aural indication of settings

7 Pull-out unit on wheels to facilitate access to microwave oven above
8 Fridge at accessible level
9 Minimum 250 mm high × 150 mm wide toe recess
10 Adequate turning space for ease of movement throughout kitchen
11 High-level units within reach and only 200 mm deep

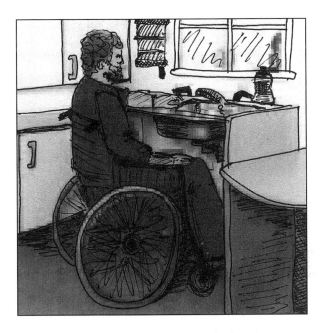

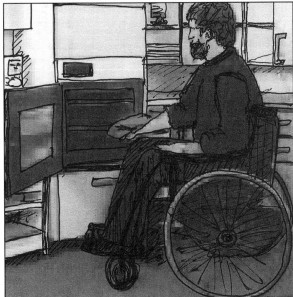

**Figure 8.11** Wheelchair user in accessible kitchen. (Reproduced with kind permission from *Buildings for Everyone*, 2002, National Disability Authority, Ireland.)

■ Locate dining and cooking areas close to each other, preferably open plan.

■ Use slip-resistant floor finish.

■ Counters to be 850 mm high generally, part at 750 mm; adjustable tops are ideal.

■ Use contrasting colours for worktops, utensils, crockery and appliance controls.

■ Provide shallow sink, convenient to cooker, with swan-neck mixer lever tap.

■ Separate oven and ceramic hob is best.

■ Use D-shaped handles on fittings.

■ Provide accessible first aid cabinet, fire blanket and fire extinguisher.

■ The zone from 450 to 1300 mm over finished floor level is the most accessible for everybody. Site all critical items in this zone.
  Provide 1500 × 1500 mm turning circle.

■ Units should have a toe recess 250 high × 150 mm deep, with knee space in key areas.

■ Carousel corner units under worktops provide the most accessible layout.

## Bathroom/shower room (Figs 8.12 and 8.13)

*Universal Design Principles:* **Equitable Use**, *Flexibility in Use*, **Low Physical Effort**, **Size and Space for Approach and Use**, *Simple and Intuitive Use, Perceptible Information, Tolerance for Error.*

The restricted space and access provision within the male WC/bathing/showering block should be altered to adhere to safe manual handling practices. Many of the cubicle doors open out into the corridor area with consequent risk of injury to others.

■ Provide minimum 400 mm wide ledge or platform at the end of the bath.

■ Bath to be 1600 mm long, 500–550 mm high (450 mm in wheelchair-accessible bathrooms), with built-in slip resistance, sloped end and lever-type taps located on inner rim.

■ Provide grabrails, 35 mm diameter.

■ Provide washbasin extending to 430–450 mm out from wall, finishing 750–800 mm over floor, fitted on brackets, within reach of WC.

■ Provide accessible mirror and towel rails.

■ Floor finish to be slip-resistant, avoid loose mats.

■ Ensure ventilation controls are accessible.

■ Provide a level-deck shower in place of a bath in wheelchair-accessible en suites.

■ Provide privacy by means of a curtain rather than rigid doors.

Accessible shower room

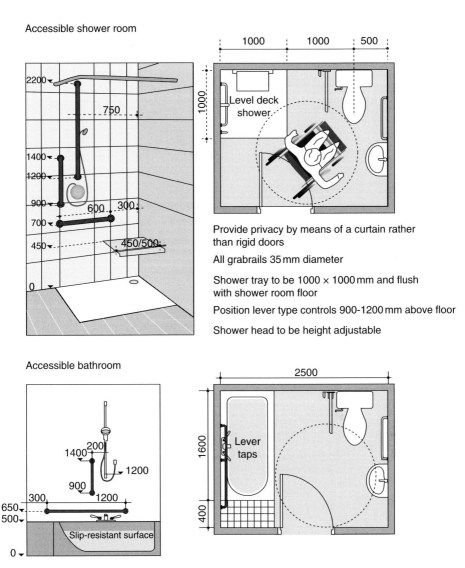

1000   1000   500

Level deck shower

Provide privacy by means of a curtain rather than rigid doors

All grabrails 35 mm diameter

Shower tray to be 1000 × 1000 mm and flush with shower room floor

Position lever type controls 900–1200 mm above floor

Shower head to be height adjustable

Accessible bathroom

2500

1600   400

Lever taps

Slip-resistant surface

**Figure 8.12** Wheelchair-accessible bath/shower in institutional setting. (Reproduced with kind permission from *Buildings for Everyone*, 2002, National Disability Authority, Ireland.)

- ▩ Shower tray to be 1000 × 1000 mm and flush with shower room floor.
- ▩ Position lever-type controls 900–1200 mm above floor.
- ▩ Provide thermostatic cut-off; the temperature of hot water in wash basins should be restricted to no more than 43°C and should be thermostatically controlled in showers. People with poor heat register are likely to be scalded if water is too hot. The same is true for people with impaired mobility, who may not be able to react quickly when scalding water issues from a tap or shower head.

Domestic bathroom –
window opposite entrance

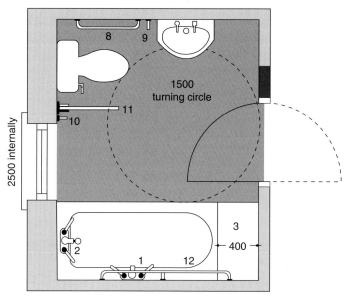

Domestic WC

**Bath and shower rooms**

**Doors**
- 800 mm clear opening width
- lever type handles with easy-to-use lock
- door frame to facilitate future reversal of swing – use pivot hinges and removable door stops; consider implications on space outside
- door to have fixing blocks 1000 mm above finished floor level (FFL) for a future 400 mm long pull handle

**WC pan**
- seat to finish 450–460 mm over FFL
- securely fix cistern lid
- flush handle to be positioned on transfer side of pan – see drawings

**Wash hand basin**
- full size wall-mounted wash hand basin to finish 750–900 mm over FFL
- use lever taps
- allow 700 mm clear knee space underneath
- within reach of WC – see Figs. 7.5, 7.7
- mirror 900–1800 mm over FFL

**Bath**
- 1600 mm long bath, 450 mm rim height
- avoid bucket or steep end baths
- use lever taps
- bath to have built in slip resistance
1 ideal position of taps
2 acceptable position of taps
3 400 mm deep ledge

**Figure 8.13** Wheelchair-accessible bath/shower in domestic setting and suitable for lifetime design. (Reproduced with kind permission from *Buildings for Everyone*, 2002, National Disability Authority, Ireland.)

Domestic bathroom –
window at right angles to entrance

2000 internally

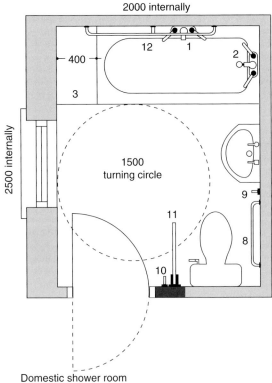

2500 internally

400

1500
turning circle

Domestic shower room

1650 internally

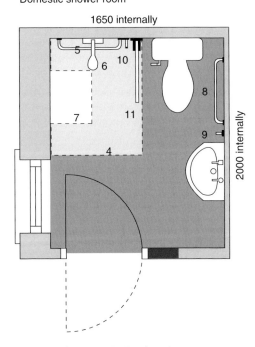

2000 internally

**Shower**
4 either lay entire floor to fall, or use a flush finish
shower tray surrounded by fabric shower curtain
5 lever controls for temperature and flow at
900–1200 mm above tray
6 shower head adjustable within range of
1200–2200 mm above tray
7 flip-up seat, 450–500 mm wide, to finish 450 mm
above tray

**Grab rails**
• generally provide only fixing blocks for future
installation of 35 mm diameter grab rails as follows:
8 horizontal grab rail 600 mm long, 700 mm above
FFL, and 200 mm from internal corner
9 vertical grab rail, 600 mm long, 200 mm from tap
centre-line, starting 700 mm above FFL
10 vertical grab rail, 600 mm long, 500 mm from
WC centre-line, starting 700 mm above FFL
11 fold-up grab rail 400 mm from WC centre-line,
700 mm from FFL
12 1200 mm long horizontal grab rail in conjunction
with 600 mm long vertical grab rail

**Floor**
• slip-resistant material. Drainage gulley is
desirable with floor finish falling towards gulley;
site gulley where it will not cause an obstruction

**Window**
• provide direct access so as to open window and
control ventilator fans

**Figure 8.13** *Continued.*

## *Toilet*

*Universal Design Principles:* **Equitable Use**, *Low Physical Effort,* **Size and Space for Approach and Use**, *Simple and Intuitive Use, Perceptible Information, Tolerance for Error, Flexibility in Use.*

The limited space and access provision within the male WC/bathing/showering block should be altered to adhere to safe manual handling practices. Many of the cubicle doors open out into the corridor area with consequent risk of injury to others. Attention needs to be given to toilet design so as to minimise the difficulties many people will have in using them.

### Standard toilet blocks

- Clear space of 1200 × 1200 mm outside all lobby and cubicle doors.
- One in six cubicles to be suitable for ambulant disabled people.
- Cubicle doors to open inwards.
- WC pan seat to be 395–410 mm over floor.
- Washbasins to finish 750–900 mm over floor.
- Taps to be lever type or automatic.
- Urinals to have 750 × 1200 mm clear approach.
- One in six urinals to be 380 mm over floor.

### Toilets for people who need assistance (Fig. 8.14)

A peninsular-type toilet is suitable for hospitals, nursing homes and other buildings with a significant occupancy of wheelchair users who need assistance to transfer. The minimum 750 mm clear unobstructed width required in the wheelchair-accessible toilet should be provided to both sides of the pan. Boxed-in cisterns should be avoided. This allows for either left- or right-handed lateral transfer and for space for an assistant at the same time. The provision of a peninsular-type toilet does not preclude the need for the standard wheelchair-accessible toilet. People who can use a wheelchair-accessible toilet independently may not be able to use a peninsular type without assistance.

### Toilets for ambulant disabled people (Fig. 8.15)

- 900 mm wide and 1800 mm long.
- Horizontal and vertical grabrails on both sides of pan.
- Standard pan – seat at 395–410 mm over floor.

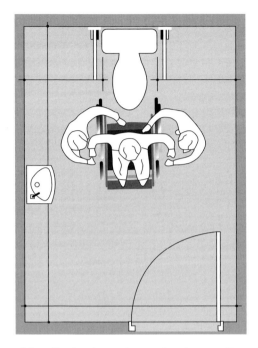

**Figure 8.14** Accessible toilet for those who need assistance. (Reproduced with kind permission from *Buildings for Everyone*, 2002, National Disability Authority, Ireland.)

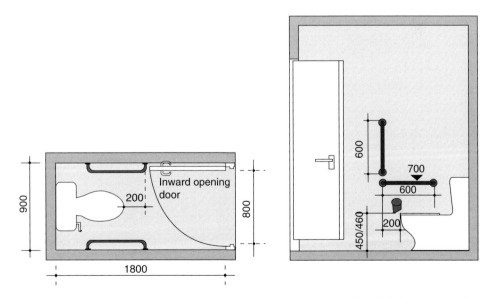

**Figure 8.15** Accessible toilet for people who are ambulant disabled. (Reproduced with kind permission from *Buildings for Everyone*, 2002, National Disability Authority, Ireland.)

### Wheelchair-accessible toilets (Fig. 8.16)

■ Cubicle to be 1500 mm wide and 2700 mm long.
■ Ensure all dimensions of space and positioning of fittings are strictly adhered to.
■ Inward opening door on short side.
■ WC seat height 450–460 mm.
■ Securely fix cistern lids to WCs.
■ Provide backrest where high-level cisterns are used.
■ Use lever-type flush handles.
■ Avoid split toilet seats.
■ Locate flush handle on transfer side in wheelchair-accessible WC.
■ Rinse basin to be 450 mm × 300 mm, and 800 mm above floor.
■ Use single mixer taps with lever or automatic operation.
■ Mirrors and coat hooks to be universally accessible.
■ Floor finish to be slip-resistant.
■ Provide easy-to-use locks.
■ Ensure sanitary fittings contrast in colour with the walls.
■ Avoid fittings with sharp edges.

## Ambient conditions

*Universal Design Principles: Equitable Use, Flexibility in Use, **Simple and Intuitive Use, Perceptible Information**, Tolerance for Error, Low Physical Effort, Size and Space for Approach and Use.*

■ Reduce glare from glazing.
■ Reduce glare from high-sheen surfaces.
■ Manage competing visual stimuli.
■ Manage competing auditory stimuli.

## Communication – hearing and vision

*Universal Design Principles: **Equitable Use**, Flexibility in Use, Simple and Intuitive Use, **Perceptible Information**, Tolerance for Error, Low Physical Effort, **Size and Space for Approach and Use**.*

### Communication systems

■ Install induction and counter loops in reception areas, meeting rooms and areas requiring confidentiality and where glazed screens affect communication.
■ Provide appropriate signs to indicate installation of induction and counter loops.

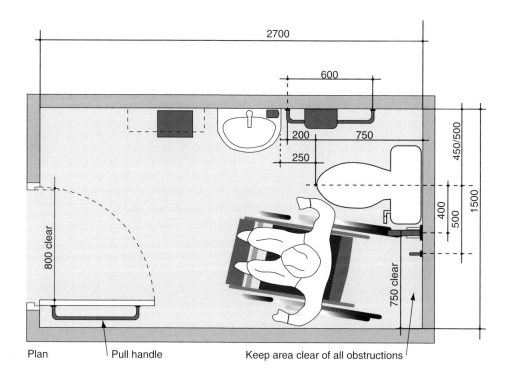

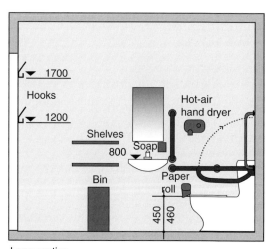

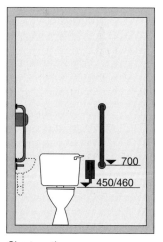

Plan     Pull handle     Keep area clear of all obstructions

Long section             Short section

**Figure 8.16** Wheelchair-accessible toilet. (Reproduced with kind permission from *Buildings for Everyone*, 2002, National Disability Authority, Ireland.)

▪ Make portable loops available for areas without permanent loop systems.
▪ Ensure that at least part of any loop system is located within 15.0 m of the person speaking.
▪ Locate doorbell controls 900–1200 mm over finished ground level.
▪ Use large bell pushes, supplemented by light to indicate use.
▪ Use combined visual/audible public address and cueing systems.

## Signs

▪ Signs to be legible by both sight and touch where appropriate.
▪ Site signs to avoid obstruction or reduced headroom.
▪ Position signs where the reader will not obstruct traffic flow.
▪ Use conventional sizes, colours and shapes.
▪ Position room numbers and names on the wall adjacent to the door handle.
▪ Provide for comfortable reading positions: tilt sign where necessary.
▪ Provide symbols to indicate services/facilities where possible.

## Lighting

*Universal Design Principles: **Equitable Use**, **Flexibility in Use**, Simple and Intuitive Use, **Perceptible Information**, Tolerance for Error, Low Physical Effort, Size and Space for Approach and Use.*

▪ Use light to express texture, colour and shape.
▪ Select appropriate light intensities for specific tasks.
▪ Position light sources to maximise distribution, minimise glare and avoid shadows.
▪ Plan stairwell and step lighting to avoid shadows.
▪ Avoid light sources which put building users in silhouette.
▪ Provide lighting controls to permit variation in light intensity.
▪ Provide blinds to permit control of natural light.
▪ Provide dimmer controls for artificial lighting.
▪ Controls should be easy to operate and located in accessible positions.
▪ Use rocker-type light switches in 20 mm deep switch housings.

## Flooring

*Universal Design Principles: Equitable Use, Flexibility in Use, Simple and Intuitive Use, Perceptible Information, Tolerance for Error, **Low Physical Effort, Size and Space for Approach and Use**.*

- Consider slip resistance, particularly if floor is likely to become wet.
- Consider ease of use for buggies and wheelchairs when selecting pile depth for carpeting; avoid deep pile carpets and coir mats.
- Consider the use of natural materials in relation to the needs of people with impaired breathing.
- Provide flush thresholds internally and externally.
- Detail matwells so that mat pile is maximum 12 mm deep and finishes flush with floor generally.
- Avoid loose mats.
- Detail floor finish, colour and texture to highlight room entrances and other significant elements or components.
- Provide colour and texture signals at tops and bottoms of all ramps and flights of stairs.
- Select non-reflective floor finishes.

## Bedrooms

*Universal Design Principles:* **Equitable Use**, *Flexibility in Use, Simple and Intuitive Use,* **Perceptible Information**, *Tolerance for Error, Low Physical Effort,* **Size and Space for Approach and Use**.

Beds should be 450 mm high to provide for easy transfer and should be height adjustable to facilitate a range of users and carers during manual handling tasks. Beds should have firm edges on the outer rim. Ensure a minimum 1500 × 1500 mm turning space (for those using mobility equipment). Provide an 800 mm zone around the bed to facilitate access and movement around the room. Plan so as to permit alternative bed positions, enabling both left- and right-hand transfer from wheelchair to bed.

King's Fund beds will be provided for each patient, which have approximate dimensions of 940 × 2190 mm. Therefore, when adhering to the above guidance, bedrooms should if possible not be less than 3300 × 2900 mm to facilitate safe transfer and provision of necessary bedroom furniture. Since rooms are not en suite it may be necessary to provide commodes for some patients from time to time so space and approach within bedrooms should facilitate dignity and safe use. More ambulant patients without continence difficulties may find rooms of 2700 × 2700 mm accessible although this will be fairly cramped accommodation.

In accessible bedroom accommodation, it is essential that users can control lights from the bed. This can be done by additional two- or three-way switching reachable from the bed, remote control operation or press-cable control switches. Pull-cord controls should be capable of operation without gripping or clasping. Avoid trailing cables and lamps with switches beside the bulbs.

### Living room/lounges/dining room/male/female areas

*Universal Design Principles:* **Equitable Use, Flexibility in Use, Simple and Intuitive Use, Perceptible Information,** *Tolerance for Error,* **Low Physical Effort, Size and Space for Approach and Use.**

As a priority, attention should be addressed to environmental cueing and flooring. Colour schemes should be devised that may assist the service user/patient to better understand and access the environment. In this way the environment is compensating for or adjusting to the patient's cognitive limitations. These areas should use colour to assist the user in identifying and locating these spaces. Upholstery drapes and wall colour can provide environmental cues to assist the user in way finding. Each area should have a different scheme, using block rather than patterned colour schemes to help orientate those with memory or other cognitive deficit. The less demanding the environmental stimulation is for the client, the more easily s/he will be able to process the information. However, if the environment is too lacking in environmental difference and detail, there will be insufficient information available to assist with orientation.

Way-finding (WCs, dining room, female area) can also be assisted by painting directional walkways/paths on walls or floors. This can include coloured route-ways to dining, WC and male/female areas within the ward. Clear signage with use of symbols can also improve orientation for those with dementia, as can the use of uni/block coloured upholstery/drapes in identifying ward areas and function of areas. As a rule, the environment should aim to cater to the needs of the lowest functioning patients as they will be unable to adapt to high-demand environments. Higher functioning patients will be able to adapt more easily as they may possess higher cognitive and sensory processing skills and increased mobility. Plain, non-patterned fabrics are less confusing for clients with dementia as they demand fewer processing skills to understand.

The furniture should be sturdy and chairs should be heavy and have arms and high backs to facilitate safe transfer. Fabric chosen for upholstery should be anti-shear.

## Universal design to support the brain

The vast majority of universal design applications tend to focus on people with physical and sensory impairments such as issues that affect mobility, reach, sensory information and energy expenditure (Calkins *et al*. 2001). These features clearly support the principles of universal design but they do not embrace it totally. Other elements must also be taken into consideration if universal design is to achieve its goal of making environments that are usable by everyone. Universal design can also support the brain by using what we know about the brain and the way it manages information about the environment (Zeisel 2001).

In Chapter 5 we saw how the environment can support (affordance) or restrict (press) occupational performance. It is the brain that enables us to understand our environment and different parts of the brain assist with this function. We know that unsupportive environments can divert mental energy from the task at hand. Noisy or overstimulating environments can lead to irritability of the user and distractions may occur, leading to difficulty with occupational performance. The converse is also true; environments that are understimulating, where there is poor fit between a person's ability and the arousal produced by the environment, can lead to boredom which may also disrupt occupational performance.

The brain is important in enabling individuals to interpret their environment; parts of the brain are involved in the task of finding one's way, remembering places and important landmarks, interpreting information and acting on this appropriately. Zeisel (2001) proposes eight fundamental environmental characteristics and their corresponding mind–brain functional areas that should be considered in environmental design for those with cognitive impairment. Calkins *et al*. (2001) further build on the seven principles of universal design to include additional guidelines that support cognition and these will be presented in detail later in this chapter.

Although the understanding of cognitive needs within environmental design can include a broad range of users, including those with mental health difficulties, the application is especially relevant for those with Alzheimer's disease. People with dementia often become anxious and agitated in new and unfamiliar areas such as institutional settings. In this distressed state, individuals can hit out at others and may also be prone to other forms of aggression. Zeisel (2001) proposes that correctly designed environments can greatly reduce these symptoms and the associated behaviour. Zeisel notes that cognitively intact people respond to environments in the same way as do those with dementia but because of their intact cognitive processes, and in particular the role of the hippocampus, which is not intact in the brains of those with dementia, they are able to control their response. Designing environments that do not evoke the responses listed above benefits a broad spectrum of users and promotes satisfactory occupational performance. By designing the environment to meet the needs of the less able, all those up to and within that ability range will be able to use that environment.

## Design principles for dementia

Calkins *et al.* (2001) identify five basic design principles that relate specifically to the cognitive limitations of individuals with dementia and although there is some congruence with the principles of universal design, there are also some differences. The design principles for dementia focus primarily on the loss of cognitive functioning, as opposed to the mainly physical and sensory functional loss which is the focus of universal design. During the course of the past two decades, research findings (Calkins *et al.* 2001) have supported a positive therapeutic approach as opposed to the earlier care approach that focused primarily on symptom management and specific functional deficits such as wandering, combativeness and agitation. The current approach is known as the person-centred therapeutic goals approach, which contains seven goals.

### 1. Awareness and orientation: the ability to know where one is in relation to where one wishes to go

This ability is affected by the structure and organisation of the environment and includes placement, design and use of signage, landmarks and other cues.

### 2. Safety and security

This is fundamental to any dementia care setting because the physical and cognitive limitations that characterise this condition can render any environment dangerous to the individual. Management of risk through the use of wandering monitoring and other automated systems, in addition to the provision of the mobility/access supports discussed earlier, will be important in this setting.

### 3. Privacy

Access to a space where individuals can be alone as a means to regulate their interaction with others. Individuals are provided with the means to control the amount of interactions with others.

## 4. Functional abilities

As the condition progresses, individuals increasingly lose the ability to perform complex tasks such as self-care and activities of daily living. A competence-inducing environment together with social supports can go some way towards meeting the individual's functional deficits. Such environments promote the continued use of everyday skills.

## 5. Personal control

Independent autonomy should be promoted whilst the individual's performance capacities allow it. This may be achieved through the environmental options offered within the setting. Access to a variety of social spaces is one example of promoting autonomy.

## 6. Continuity of self

As the condition progresses one's sense of self and memory of self diminish. Loss of identity is the experience for many with the consequent associated behavioural changes. The environmental application of this goal promotes the personalisation and familiarisation of environments that contain elements from the person's past, thus providing a context or frame of reference for their behaviour.

## 7. Social contact

As the condition progresses, language skills and executive functioning skills are lost, which detrimentally affects interaction skills. Initiating and sustaining conversations with others become difficult. An environment that provides social supports will offer opportunities (affordance) for individuals to practise these skills.

These person-based goals are supported by the following five principles of dementia design and their guidelines.

## 1. Minimal negative sensation: harmonious environments free from excessive and competing stimuli

This principle is based on the ecology model that establishes a relationship between the demands of the environment (press) and the individual's performance capacities. Negative stimulation can cause stress which may in turn lead to behavioural difficulties such as aggression and agitation.

- *Reduce scale.* Smaller environments support the goals of awareness and orientation, functional abilities, social contact and safety and security.
- *Control ambient conditions.* Remove distracting auditory and visual background stimuli (paging systems, busy wallpaper and upholstery patterns, glare, television, etc.). Supports the goals of awareness and orientation, functional abilities, social contact.
- *Limit choices.* Reduce the complexity of decision making but do not remove choices altogether as this can have a detrimental effect on behaviour. Too many choices can be confusing and stressful for individuals with dementia and so should therefore be limited to a few meaningful options (clothing selections, menu, etc.). Supports the goals of functional abilities and personal control.
- *Provide place for retreat.* Enables the overwhelmed individual to leave a stressful/overstimulating situation. Supports the goals of privacy and personal control.

### 2. Maximal positive stimulation: supportive environment that adjusts to meet functional demands

This principle is based on the ecology model that establishes a relationship between the supports of the environment (affordance) and the individual's performance capacities.

- *Augmentative cues.* Promotes full sensory experiences through the use of augmentative cues to help orientate individuals to time and place (visual, auditory or olfactory cues are commonly used). Supports the goal of functional abilities.
- *Focusing.* Refers to guiding attention to the most important environmental elements through design. One example of this would be to highlight the location of WCs or other key environmental features by using colour to differentiate from surrounding environment, place in prominent and central position determined by the activity, desired outcome and the social gathering points of the unit. Supports the goals of functional abilities and social contact.
- *Non-standardisation.* Avoid the use of repeated patterns, colours and spaces. The focus is to enable way finding by providing differentiation. This can be achieved through the use of bright colours, landmarks and prominent signage. Supports the goals of awareness and orientation, functional abilities, personal control, and continuity of self.

### 3. Familiarity: the environment facilitates and reminds individuals of real-life patterns based upon the assumption of the endurance of long-term memory

- *Non-institutional imagery.* Institutional environments are not part of an individual's past daily experience and so care must be taken to use imagery that is familiar to individuals. The absence of such familiarity can lead to stress and aggressive outbursts. Imagery from domestic settings is a common successful application. Supports the goals of awareness and orientation and continuity of self.
- *Public to private spatial continuum.* This guideline is closely linked to the preceding one and relates to organisational layout of domestic spaces. In most homes the public spaces (lounges, etc.) are located close to the entrance of the home whilst the more private spaces (bedrooms, etc.) are located further within the structure. Care settings should aim to replicate this arrangement. The absence of such awareness and provision can lead to stress, confusion and aggressive outbursts. Supports the goals of personal control, privacy and continuity of self.
- *Reduced learning.* Use artefacts, signs and symbols that are (as safely as possible) familiar to the individual. Wherever possible, the environment should not impose new learning on the individual. To assist with way finding, simple clear signs or pictures can be used to offer familiarity. Supports the goals of awareness and orientation, functional abilities and continuity of self.

### 4. Continuity: the environment supports the past patterns of a person's life and offers opportunities to express these

This principle relates to but goes beyond the principle of familiarity as it relates directly to each individual in the setting.

- *Personalisation.* Promotes the meaningful use of artefacts from a person's past. Individuals are encouraged to display photos, meaningful personal objects, etc. in their bedrooms. Supports the goals of awareness and orientation, personal control and continuity of self.
- *Recreating past patterns and places.* Promotes the recreation of past work, domestic and recreational patterns. Examples include opportunities for assisting with laundry or baking in the therapeutic kitchen or perhaps opportunities for assisting in office or gardening activities if these are meaningful to individuals. Supports the goals of continuity of self, functional abilities and social contact.

**Table 8.1** Relationship between universal design and dementia design principles. (Adapted from Calkins *et al.* 2001. Permission for use of this information has been granted by MacGraw-Hill.)

| Dementia design principles and guidance ↓ / Universal design principles and guidance → | Equitable Use — Provide same means of use for all users – identical when possible, equivalent when not | Flexibility in Use — Provide choice in methods of use, accommodate right- or left-handed use; facilitate user's accuracy and precision | Simple and Intuitive Use — Eliminate complexity; be consistent with expectations and intuition; provide effective prompting of sequential actions and timely feedback | Perceptible Information — Use redundant presentation; contrast between information and surroundings; maximise legibility | Tolerance for Error — Make most used elements most accessible, isolate, eliminate or shield hazards; discourage unconscious actions | Low Physical Effort — Allow user to maintain natural body positions, use reasonable operating forces, minimise repetitive actions and sustained physical effort | Size and Space for Approach and Use — Provide adequate space for reach, manipulation, use and assistance; provide clear line of sight, accommodate variation in hand and grip size |
|---|---|---|---|---|---|---|---|
| **Minimal Negative Sensation** | | | | | | | |
| Reduce scale | | | | | | | I |
| Control ambient conditions | | | E | | | | |
| Limit choices | | | | | | | |
| Provide place for retreat | C | | | C | | | I |
| **Maximal Positive Stimulation** | | | | | | | |
| Augmentative cues | | | | I | | | |
| Focusing | | | | E | | | |
| Non-standardisation | | | | I | | | |
| **Familiarity** | | | | | | | |
| Non-institutional imagery | | | I | | | | |
| Public to private continuum | | C | I | | | | |
| Reduced learning | C | C | C | | | C | |
| **Continuity** | | | | | | | |
| Personalisation | I | | | | | | |
| Familiar patterns | I | | | | | | |
| Individualised cueing | I | I | | | | | |
| **Regulated Access** | | | | | | | |
| Selective access | C | C | C | C | I | C | C |
| Sheilded hazardous elements | C | C | C | C | I | C | C |
| Supervision | C | C | C | C | I | C | I |

C, contradiction between universal design and dementia design; I, implicit in or compatible with universal design principle; E, explicitly stated in universal design principle.

▪ *Individualised cueing.* Multisensory cueing should be based on familiar past patterns and experience. Olfactory cues help remind the person that it's time to eat; also some cultures traditionally eat certain foods on particular days, for example eating fish on Friday can help to orientate to time. Supports the goals of awareness and orientation, functional abilities and continuity of self.

### 5. Regulated access: the environment controls, limits or facilitates the monitoring of access to potential hazards

▪ *Selective access.* Access to hazardous elements is determined by cognitive function and abilities. Examples include using complicated locks and providing boundaries around safe territory (e.g. garden). The provision of care staff to support individuals as condition progresses is also included within this principle (e.g. assisted toileting). Supports the goals of safety and security and functional abilities.

▪ *Shielding hazardous elements.* This relates to using the individual's deficits to create barriers to hazardous areas and objects. An example is the camouflage of hazardous elements such as doors leading to unsafe places to discourage use whilst those leading to safe and desired places are highlighted for facilitated access and use. Another example is the use of lowered beds to prevent night-time wandering and reduce the incidence of falls. Supports the goal of safety and security.

▪ *Supervision.* The arrangement of space and plans (discussed in earlier sections of this chapter) strongly supports or inhibits the ability of carers to care for individuals with cognitive, sensory and physical impairments. The use of technology such as wander monitoring and bed occupancy systems helps with implementing this guideline. Supports the goal of safety and security.

Table 8.1 illustrates the relationship between dementia design and universal design. By using both design principles in the dementia setting, a more holistic and comprehensive design perspective guides the practitioner in the environmental adjustment process for this population.

## References

Calkins M, Sanford J, Proffitt M (2001) Design for dementia: challenges and lessons for universal design. In: Preiser W, Ostroff E (eds) *Universal Design Handbook.* McGraw-Hill, New York.

Iwarsson S, Isacsson Å (1996) Development of a novel instrument for occupational therapy assessment of the physical environment in the home – a methodologic study on 'The Enabler'. *Occupational Therapy Journal of Research* **16(4)**, 227–244.

National Disability Authority (NDA) (2002) *Buildings for Everyone: inclusion, access and use*. National Disability Authority, Dublin, Ireland.

Zeisel J (2001) Universal design to support the brain and its development. In: Preiser W, Ostroff E (eds) *Universal Design Handbook*. McGraw-Hill, New York.

# PART 3
# The Sociopolitical Context

'In twenty years, men may be able to live on the Moon. In forty years we may get to Mars. In the next 200 years we may leave the solar system and head for the stars. But meanwhile, we would like to get to the supermarket, the cinema, restaurants' (Hawkings 2007).

# 9: The sociopolitical environment: policy

The words on the previous page by Professor Stephen Hawking, one of the greatest scientific minds of our time and also an individual with significant physical impairment, strike at the core of the issue. We humans have not only managed to push forward the boundaries of our known world but we are forging ahead into the unexplored regions of the universe. The technology, resources, knowledge and will to achieve these exploratory ends are well within our grasp and yet the demands of so many individuals with impairments remain unmet, demands which far from being 'out of this world' could be met relatively easily and with benefit to society at large.

Policy, legislation and guidance are one way to influence change and can serve as a vehicle to challenge prevailing attitudes.

## The standard rules of the United Nations on the equality of opportunities for people with disabilities

In 1993 the General Assembly of the UN adopted the Standard Rules of the United Nations on the Equality of Opportunities for People with Disabilities. This document is the main reference for the universal rights of people with disabilities (Seelman 2001). It is against this document that member states determine their own policies' compliance. The document addresses accessibility in the physical environment and access to information and communication.

## International classification of functioning, disability and health

The *International Classification of Functioning, Disability and Health*, known more commonly as ICF, is a classification of the health components of functioning and disability.

After nine years of international revision efforts co-ordinated by the World Health Organization (WHO), the World Health Assembly on

May 22, 2001, approved the *International Classification of Functioning, Disability and Health* and its abbreviation of ICF. This classification was first created in 1980 (then called the *International Classification of Impairments, Disabilities and Handicaps,* or ICIDH) by the WHO to provide a unifying framework for classifying the health components of functioning and disability.

The ICF classification complements the WHO's *International Classification of Diseases,*10th revision (ICD), which contains information on diagnosis and health condition but not functional status. The ICD and ICF constitute the core classifications in the WHO family of international classifications (WHO-ICF).

The ICF is so named because its focus is on health and functioning rather than on disability. This is a radical shift. From emphasising people's disabilities, the framework now focuses on their level of health. The ICF puts the notions of 'health' and 'disability' in a new light. It acknowledges that every human being can suffer a decrement in health and thereby experience some disability. This is not something that happens to only a minority of people. The ICF thus 'mainstreams' disability and recognises it as a universal human experience.

### The ICF model

Two major conceptual models of disability have been proposed. The medical model views disability as a feature of the person, directly caused by disease, trauma or other health condition, which requires medical care provided in the form of individual treatment by professionals. Disability, in this model, calls for medical or other treatment or intervention, to 'correct' the problem. The social model, on the other hand, sees disability as a socially created problem and not at all an attribute of an individual. In the social model, disability demands a political response, since the problem is created by an unaccommodating physical environment brought about by attitudes and other features of the social environment (WHO 2002).

On their own, neither model is adequate, although both are partially valid. Disability is a complex phenomenon that is both a problem at the level of a person's body and a complex and primarily social phenomenon. Disability is always an interaction between features of the person and features of the overall context in which the person lives, but some aspects of disability are almost entirely internal to the person, while others are almost entirely external. In other words, both medical and social responses are appropriate to the problems associated with disability; we cannot wholly reject either kind of intervention. A better model of disability, in short, is one that synthesises what is true in the medical and social models, without making the mistake of reducing the whole, complex notion of disability to one of its aspects. This more useful model of disability might be called the biopsychosocial model. The ICF is based on this model, an integration of the medical and the social.

## How can the ICF be used?

Because of its flexible framework, the detail and completeness of its classifications and the fact that each domain is operationally defined, with inclusions and exclusions, it is expected that the ICF, like its predecessor, will be used to answer a wide range of questions involving clinical, research and policy development issues (WHO 2002).

The ICF is structured around the following broad components.

▪ Body functions and structure
▪ Activities (related to tasks and actions by an individual) and participation (involvement in a life situation)
▪ Additional information on severity and environmental factors (WHO 2002)

## Uses of environment factors

One of the major innovations in the ICF is the presence of an environmental factor classification that allows the identification of environmental barriers and facilitators for both capacity and performance of actions and tasks in daily living. With this classification scheme, which can be used either on an individual basis or for population-wide data collection, it may be possible to create instruments that assess environments in terms of their facilitation or barrier creation for different kinds and levels of disability. With this information in hand, it will then be more practical to develop and implement guidelines for universal design and other environmental regulations that extend the functioning of people with disabilities across the range of life activities (WHO 2001).

## Council of Europe Action Plan

The Council of Europe Disability Action Plan (2006) for 2006–2015 seeks to translate the aims of the Council of Europe with regard to human rights, non-discrimination, equal opportunities, full citizenship and participation of people with disabilities into a European policy framework on disability for the next decade. This action plan aims to provide a comprehensive framework that is both flexible and adaptable in order to meet country-specific conditions. It is intended to serve as a roadmap for policy makers, to enable them to design, adjust, refocus and implement appropriate plans, programmes and innovative strategies. The Council of Europe will seek to implement the Disability Action Plan by providing assistance to all member states in the form of recommendations, advice and expert information.

Employment and the environment are key elements for the social inclusion and economic independence of all citizens of working age. Compared to non-disabled persons, the employment and activity rates of disabled people are very low. Vocational guidance and assistance play an important role in helping people to identify activities for which they are best suited and to guide training needs or future occupation. It is vital that people with disabilities have access to assessments, vocational guidance and training to ensure they can attain their potential (Employers' Forum on Disability 2007).

This action plan for employment is intended to form the basis for greater participation of people with disabilities in employment, to ensure career choices and to lay the foundations through structures and support in order to ensure real choices. Social enterprises (for example, social firms, social co-operatives), as part of the open employment, have been recommended for further development and expansion.

## Legislation and guidance in the UK

### Disability discrimination act (DDA) 1995, amendment 2004

#### Definition of disability

A person has a disability for the purposes of the DDA if s/he has a physical or mental impairment which has a substantial and long-term adverse effect on his or her ability to carry out normal day-to-day activities.

Part 1 of the Act addresses the definition of disability and provides information and guidance on what constitutes disability for the purposes of the Act, and who is protected under it.

Part 2 addresses employment and prohibits discrimination in relation to employment of disabled people, including recruitment, training, promotion, benefits, dismissal, etc. It requires employers to make 'reasonable adjustments' for a disabled person put at a substantial disadvantage by a provision, criterion or practice, or a physical feature of premises. It also prohibits discrimination by trade organisations and qualifications bodies. It provides procedures for enforcement and provision of remedies for discrimination.

**Part 3** covers provision of goods, facilities and services, disposal or management of premises or land. Private clubs are included within Part 3. It requires service providers to make 'reasonable adjustments' for disabled people. A service provider is required to take reasonable steps to:

- change a practice, policy or procedure which makes it impossible or unreasonably difficult for disabled people to make use of its services
- provide an auxiliary aid or service if it would enable (or make it easier for) disabled people to make use of its services.

In addition, where a physical feature makes it impossible or unreasonably difficult for disabled people to make use of services, a service provider has to take reasonable steps to:

- remove the feature; or
- alter it so that it no longer has that effect; or
- provide a reasonable means of avoiding it; or
- provide a reasonable alternative method of making the service available.

It prohibits discrimination by private clubs. It provides procedures for enforcement and provision of remedies for discrimination.

**Part 4** addresses education and the 2001 Amendment to the Act prohibits discrimination in relation to:

- school admissions, exclusions and the education or associated services provided to pupils
- further and higher education admissions, exclusions and student services.

Responsible bodies for schools and further and higher education institutions must make reasonable adjustments to ensure that disabled pupils or students (or prospective pupils or students) are not placed at a substantial disadvantage in comparison with their non-disabled peers.

Responsible bodies for further and higher education are also required to provide auxiliary aids or services and have a duty to make adjustments to physical features. This Part provides procedures for enforcement and provision of remedies for discrimination.

**Part 5** addresses transport. It provides the Secretary of State with powers to establish minimum access criteria for public transport vehicles to be phased in over time. The use of transport was excluded from the requirements of Part 3 of the Act until December 2006.

**Part 6** provided for the National Disability Council which was set up to advise the Government on Parts 2 and 3 of the DDA. It was abolished when the Disability Rights Commission came into operation in April 2000.

**Part 7** deals with supplementary issues and details duties and responsibilities covering:

- codes of practice
- victimisation
- liability of employers
- help for people suffering discrimination
- aiding unlawful acts
- exclusion for acts done with statutory authority or done for the purpose of safeguarding national security.

**Part 8** deals with miscellaneous issues, including government appointments, regulations and interpretation.

**Schedules 1–8** are assorted schedules containing, among other things, provisions relating to the meaning of disability (Schedule 1), relevance of past disabilities (Schedule 2) and listing of responsible bodies for schools and educational institutions (Schedules 4A and 4B).

## Disability equality duty

The Disability Discrimination Act 2005 amended the previous Act to insert the disability equality duty, known as the general duty, into the Act. The duty is aimed at tackling systemic discrimination and ensuring that public authorities build disability equality into everything that they do (DRC 2006).

## The disability rights commission (DRC)

The Disability Rights Commission (DRC) is an independent body established in April 2000 by Act of Parliament to stop discrimination and promote equality of opportunity for disabled people.

### What the DRC does

- Gives advice and information to disabled people, employers and service providers.
- Supports disabled people in getting their rights under the DDA.
- Helps solve problems, often without going to a court or employment tribunal.
- Supports legal cases to test the limits of the law.
- Provides an independent Disability Conciliation Service for disabled people and service providers through Mediation UK.

- Campaigns to strengthen the law.
- Organises campaigns to change policy, practice and awareness.
- Produces policy statements and research on disability issues, and publications on rights and good practice for disabled people, employers and service providers (DRC 2006).

The government has announced a discrimination law review, looking towards producing a Single Equalities Act (SEA), which would apply to six dimensions of equality (religion, race, gender, age, sexuality and disability). The review is likely to set the legal framework for the next generation of equality law. Any change to the definition of the DDA would be introduced as part of a Single Equality Act, and the timescale is likely to be about 2010 (DRC 2006).

One of the most distinctive features of the DDA, compared to other equality laws, is that it only provides protection for a discrete and tightly defined section of the population. Other antidiscrimination laws are 'even-handed' in that they provide protection for anyone in the population if it is 'on the grounds of' race, gender, sexual orientation or religion. Men have the same degree of protection as women, for example.

There has been widespread dissatisfaction amongst disability action groups and others concerning the definition of disability contained within the DDA on the basis that it is derived from the medical model. Many now seek to broaden that definition so that the law provides protection against discrimination on the grounds of impairment, regardless of level or type of impairment. Such a change would move the disability discrimination law closer to, but not identical with, the approach of other discrimination laws. The chief advantage of such a change to the definition would be to shift the focus of attention from the medical condition of an individual to a consideration of whether or not discrimination is occurring (DRC 2006).

An EU Directive in 2000 prohibited discrimination 'on the grounds' of disability. The Directive did not define disability. It is likely that the European Court of Justice will be asked to develop, probably through a piecemeal approach, a European definition.

## Built environment legislation and development policy UK

### Chronically sick and disabled persons act 1970

This was the first piece of legislation to refer to access to the built environment for disabled people. The Act clearly states that premises open to the public, whether on payment or otherwise, should make provision for disabled visitors. Educational buildings and local authorities with reference to publicly owned housing are also to make provision.

### Town and country planning act 1990

Section 76 of the Town and Country Planning Act 1990 requires that, when granting planning permission, local planning authorities draw the attention of developers to the relevant sections of the Chronically Sick and Disabled Persons Act 1970 and to design guidance published by the BSI and the Department of Education and Science on access issues, namely BS 5810:1979 Code of Practice for Access for the Disabled to Buildings and Design Note 18 (1984) Access for Disabled People to Educational Buildings.

### Planning policy guidance note 1 (PPG1)

The most recent government advice for planning authorities appeared in the form of PPG 1, revised in February 1997. This states that:

'Proposals for the development of land provide the opportunity to secure a more accessible environment for everyone, including wheelchair users, other people with disabilities, elderly people and those with young children. Local planning authorities, both in development plans and in determining individual planning applications, should take into account access issues. These will include access to and into buildings, and the need for accessible housing.'

The internal layout of buildings is not normally material to the consideration of planning permission. Part M of Schedule 1 to the Building Regulations 1991 imposes requirements on how non-domestic buildings should be designed and constructed to secure specific objectives for people with disabilities. It would be inappropriate to use planning legislation to impose separate requirements in these areas.

When a new building is proposed, or when planning permission is required for the alteration or change of use of an existing building, the developer and local planning authority should consider the needs of people with disabilities at an early stage in the design process. They should be flexible and imaginative in seeking solutions, taking account of the particular circumstance of each case.

Resolving problems by negotiation will always be preferable but where appropriate, the planning authority may impose conditions requiring access provisions for people with disabilities.

### The building regulations

Part M of the Building Regulations 1999, 'Access and facilities for disabled people', requires reasonable provision for disabled people be made to all new dwellings, public buildings and some defined extensions (ODPM 2006). The design guidance detailed in this document sets out standards of accessibility which in some places go beyond minimum standards detailed in the Building Regulations for achieving reasonable provision. However, in light of the publication of BS 8300 2001: Design of buildings and their approaches to meet the needs of disabled people – Code of practice, further revisions to Part M (1999 Edition) of the Building Regulations were included in the 2003 amendment. The amendments relate to the duty on all service providers to make reasonable adjustments under the provisions of the DDA. Service providers are required to take reasonable steps to remove, alter or provide a reasonable means of avoiding a physical feature on their premises that renders difficult or impossible the use of their service by disabled people (ODPM 2006).

## BS 8300 2001: design of buildings and their approaches to meet the needs of disabled people – code of practice

The BSI has published a new code of practice on accessible design to explain how the built environment can be designed to anticipate, and overcome, restrictions relating to access that many disabled people encounter. The document covers a wide range of disabilities and different types of buildings including homes, retail, employment, sports venues and theatres.

The British Standard is a source of best practice for architects, builders and facilities managers and encourages innovative design solutions. Reference should be made to this comprehensive BS in addition to this publication.

BSI guidelines published in 1978 entitled 'Code of practice for the design of housing for the convenience of disabled people', BS 5619 and BS 5810 published the following year have all been superseded by BS 8300.

## Joseph Rowntree Foundation Lifetime Homes

In 1991 the Lifetime Homes concept was developed by a group of housing experts who came together as the Joseph Rowntree Foundation Lifetime Homes Group. Lifetime Homes have 16 design features that ensure that a new house or flat will meet the needs of most households.

There have been substantial developments in access standards for new-build housing. Lifetime Homes have been implemented in the UK since1997. The Joseph Rowntree Foundation is one of the largest social policy research and development charities in the UK (Sangster 1997).

## Buildings for Everyone

The publication *Buildings for Everyone* (2001), published by the National Disability Authority (NDA) of Ireland, is an excellent design guide. It introduces the concept of universal access to buildings and the external environment, outlines the principles on which Building for Everyone is based and offers clear guidance on how to achieve universal access in relation to physical and sensory impairment (NDA 2002). It shows the consequences for design and management of considering the broad range of ability and outlines the role and contribution of the various professions and agencies which are involved in shaping the built environment.

## The EC and international legislation and guidance

In 2000 the European Community (EC) enacted two laws (or in EC terminology, directives) that prevent people in the European Union from being discriminated against on grounds of race and ethnic origin (Racial Equality Directive) and on grounds of religion or belief, disability, age or sexual orientation (Employment Framework Directive). The two directives define a set of principles that offer all EU citizens a common minimum level of legal protection against discrimination (Albrecht *et al.* 2001). They follow directly from Article 13 of the Treaty establishing the EC and were unanimously agreed by the EU governments within 18 months of the Treaty of Amsterdam, entering into force in May 1999.

All EU member states were due to have transposed the directives into national laws by the end of 2003. However, this process has not been uniformly applied in the EU countries. For those that did not meet the deadlines for compliance, and had not requested an extension period, the European Community has now initiated infringement procedures to ensure that transposition occurs (Albrecht *et al.* 2001).

Whilst most EU countries have now introduced disability discrimination laws, generally these are fairly recent and are untested by case law or in practice. A wide range of approaches to definition has been adopted (DRC 2006).

## Belgium

The Belgian Act to Combat Discrimination does not define disability, on the basis that any definition would result in an exclusion of that which was not mentioned. However, the parliamentary discussion did make it clear that the intention was to interpret the concept of disability very broadly. Some commentators argued that, given this intention, it would have been more appropriate to have included a definition, or legislative guidance, on this point so as to ensure that the term 'disability' was not interpreted in the way common in daily use (DRC 2006).

## Holland

The Dutch Act on Equal Treatment on grounds of Disability or Chronic Illness (2003) also does not provide a definition of disability. The legislation covers discrimination on the grounds of 'a real or supposed disability or chronic illness' (DRC 2006).

## Finland: constitutional reform

The Disabled Persons Equality Act 1987 (Services and Assistance for the Disabled) aims to improve the ability of the disabled person to live and act as a member of society in equality with others. It has often resulted in inequalities depending upon which region people live in. Although the provision of certain services (transport and accommodation) is a right, other services are dependent on municipality funds and how they organise their services (Albrecht *et al.* 2001).

The Act on the Status and Rights of Patients (1992) is the only one which has a clear antidiscrimination clause regarding health-care provision.

In August 1995, the Constitution Act was amended (1995) to include and alter clauses regarding the fundamental rights of the citizen to directly protect the rights of disabled people and brought the Finnish system into line with international human rights conventions.

Since 1995 a clause (Chapter 11 Section 9) has been added under which it is punishable to discriminate within the course of economic/ professional activity, public service, civil service or any other public duty or in organisation of a public amusement or a public meeting lacking acceptable cause.

Employment is covered separately (Chapter 47 Section 3). Unlawful labour discrimination is found if, during the selection procedure, applicants for employment are discriminated against because of their state of health, for example. This action is punishable by fine or imprisonment (up to six months).

The social rights of citizens were adopted in the Constitution alongside traditional civil and political rights which include equal opportunities in all areas, i.e. health, education, housing. The rights of people using sign language are guaranteed by law. These rights are directly applicable for disabled people and as a prohibition of discrimination is now included in the Penal Code, it may have greater influence on courts and authorities.

### France

French law (1990, modified 1992) establishes protection for disabled persons from any discrimination they may suffer in their daily life. It prohibits discrimination by public authorities, private individuals and when being hired or dismissed. It also contains provision for advocate associations to associate themselves in a court action in cases of discrimination, with the authorisation of the interested party.

Discrimination is included in the chapter covering 'attacks on personal dignity'. Discrimination against disabled people is not specifically defined. 'Handicaps' is mentioned as a basis for discrimination along with race, sex, etc., but no special legislation covers disability.

The Penal Code introduced the principle of a 'legal persons' penal responsibility into French law which means that they can be sanctioned if found to be discriminatory by the refusal to provide goods and services, obstructing a normal economic activity or defining an offer of employment or dismissal subject to a person's handicap.

Another article of the Penal Code, however, allows discrimination in insurance, and a refusal to employ someone on the basis of an established medical condition is also not prohibited.

### Germany: antidiscrimination clause in the constitution

Article 3 of the 'Grundgesetz' sets out a non-discrimination and equal opportunity clause which states that: 'All human beings are equal before the law. Men and women have equal rights. There shall be no discrimination based on gender, birth, race, native or social origin, beliefs, religious belief or political opinion. Nobody shall be discriminated against because of disability'. This last sentence was added by the Bundestag in 1994 following lobbying by disability groups. The government's social care policy changed to one of civil rights.

The clause binds federal and state legislation and must be considered in legal cases. One of the consequences of this clause is that in some new public transport acts at state level, similar clauses were included (The Bremen Act 1995; Albrecht *et al.* 2001). The needs of users with mobility problems have to be taken into account in the buying of vehicles and in constructing any kind of traffic system, buildings and other transport facilities accessed by the public.

Discussion in Germany since 1995 has centred on an equal rights act which would change all the different areas of legislation which have had an effect on the human and civil rights of disabled people. Anti-discrimination legislation may now be operational.

## Norway

The Discrimination and Accessibility Act 2007 relates to prohibition of discrimination on the basis of disability. The legislation is characterised by the general application of protection against discrimination to most areas of society but is limited to protection in relation to a single ground of discrimination or a number of closely related grounds. The approach is based on group rights. Historically, such legislation often comes into being when a group has long been oppressed or discriminated against. After attaining a degree of strength, such groups take up the fight for better legal protection of the group. In many countries, this approach is associated with the fight for civil rights (Norwegian Report 2005). The Norwegian Gender Equality Act belongs to this category.

In other countries too there are examples of legislation against discrimination on the basis of disability that fall into this category In the USA, the UK and at the federal level in Australia, separate statutes protect against discrimination on the basis of disability, while other statutes provide protection against discrimination on the basis of gender and ethnicity. Such a broad group approach is clearly similar to the approach that has been adopted in Norway (Norwegian Report 2005).

When interpreting the prohibition against discrimination, the purpose provision in Section 1, first paragraph, has significance as an interpretive factor. This is worded as follows: 'The purpose of the Act is to ensure equality and promote equal opportunities for social participation for all persons regardless of functional ability and to prevent discrimination on the basis of disability'.

Section 11 lays down clear obligations that 'buildings, constructions and developed outdoor areas intended for the use of the general public' shall be subject to universal design from specified dates. These dates are not the same for new and existing buildings, etc. The date for enforcement in relation to new buildings, etc. has been set at 1 January 2009. Buildings, etc. erected or completed following major alterations (general renovation) and that are designed for the use of the general public shall, after this date, be subject to universal design. In the case of buildings, constructions and developed outdoor areas completed prior to this date and intended for the use of the general public, the requirement regarding universal design commences on 1 January 2019 (Norwegian Report 2005).

### Ireland

The Irish laws prohibiting disability discrimination (alongside discrimination on other grounds) is a constitutional prohibition and an indication of how they operate in practice. Ireland's legislation is common to a number of grounds for discrimination and covers most areas of society (DRC 2006, NDA 2002, Norwegian Report 2005). The Employment Equality Act 1998 and Equal Status Act 2000 both define disability as:

- 'the total or partial absence of a person's bodily or mental functions, including the absence of a part of a person's body, or
- the presence in the body of organisms causing, or likely to cause, chronic disease or illness, or
- the malfunction, malformation or disfigurement of a part of a person's body, or
- a condition or malfunction which results in a person learning differently from a person without the condition or malfunction, or
- a condition, disease or illness which affects a person's thought processes, perception of reality, emotions or judgement or which results in disturbed behaviour.'

The Act also states that it shall be 'taken to include a disability which exists at present, or which previously existed but no longer exists or which may exist in the future or which is imputed to a person'. Discrimination by association is also covered (DRC 2006).

### Spain

In contrast, the Spanish 'law for equal opportunities, non-discrimination and universal accessibility for disabled persons', excellent in many other ways, states that 'disabled persons shall include all those who have a grade of handicap of 33 per cent or above', linking the definition to welfare benefits law. This definition is being challenged as overly restrictive before the European Court of Justice (DRC 2006).

## Sweden

Sweden has three laws prohibiting discrimination, one of the grounds cited being disability. The first, the Prohibition of Discrimination in Working Life of People with Disability Act, was adopted in 1999. This was followed in 2002 by the Act on Equal Treatment of Students at Universities and in 2003 by the Prohibition of Discrimination Act, which applies among other things to trading in goods and services (Norwegian Report 2005).

Sweden shows a commitment to a high level of social welfare and recently adopted a number of measures to improve the situation of disabled people. Disabled people have the right to personal assistance. The Work Environment Act ensures that employers adapt the physical environment to suit the needs of the functionally disabled. Local authorities are required to plan with the aim that everyone has a home to meet their needs.

The definition of disability in Swedish policy adheres to the social model approach. The Disability Ombudsman was established in 1994, whose role is to monitor proposed non-discrimination legislation should this be enacted. The Disability Ombudsman:

- works towards improvements in legislation
- initiates discussions with authorities and organisations and uses publicity in order to prevent discriminatory treatment of disabled people
- submits an annual report to the government about issues affecting disabled people (Norwegian Report 2005).

## USA

The Americans with Disabilities Act 1990 (ADA) contains a definition which has proved in practice to be narrower than the UK's definition:

(a) physical or mental impairment that **substantially** limits one or more of the major life activities of such individuals
(b) **a record of** such an impairment (this means 'has a history of, or has been misclassified as having a mental or physical impairment that substantially limits one or more of the major life activities')
(c) being **regarded as** having such an impairment.

This is broadly similar to the British definition's approach. It has, however, been interpreted by the US courts in a much more restrictive fashion and is widely credited with undermining the policy intention behind the otherwise seminal ADA (Albrecht *et al.* 2001, DRC 2006).

## Australia

The definition of disability in the Australian Disability Discrimination Act 1992 (DDA) is the model for the Irish legislation and is identical with it. The Productivity Commission (established by the Australian government to improve laws) produced a *Review of the Disability Discrimination Act 1992* in 2004. The Commission expressly contrasted the Australian Act's definition with the UK definition (DRC 2006, Norwegian Report 2005). It noted that the UK law had taken up significant legal resources in identifying who is disabled, and contrasted this with the Australian focus on whether a discriminatory act has occurred. The report cited only one significant case regarding the coverage of the definition of disability. In Purvis v State of NSW (Department of Education and Training) 2003 the High Court of Australia ruled that 'disturbed behaviour' that is a consequence of a disability is part of the disability for the purposes of the DDA.

Much of the global policy reviewed above is responding to the needs of individuals with impairments by recognising the impact of the environment as an enabler or inhibitor of occupational performance. It is encouraging to witness the development of policies that embrace the universal design approach to inclusion. The author is hopeful that as a deeper awareness arises of the denial of basic human rights to a vulnerable section of the global community, the injustice experienced by many is finally beginning to be rectified. A promising and enriching future beckons.

## References

Albrecht GL, Seelman KD, Bury M (eds) (2001) *Handbook of Disability Studies.* Sage Publications, California.

Council of Europe Action Plan (2006) Report to promote the rights and full participation of people with disabilities in society: improving the quality of life of people with disabilities in Europe from 2006–2015. Available at: www.coe.int/T/E/Social_Cohesion/soc-sp/Integration/.

Disability Rights Commission (2006) Home page. Available at: www.DRC.org (accessed July 2007).

Employers' Forum on Disability (2007) Available at: www.employers-forum.co.uk/www/index.htm (accessed July 2007).

Hawkings S (2007) Available at: www.aisrael.org (accessed May 2007).

National Disability Authority (NDA) (2002) *Buildings for Everyone: inclusion, access and use.* National Disability Authority, Dublin, Ireland.

Norwegian Report (2005) Available at: www.odin.dep.no (accessed July 2007).

Office of the Deputy Prime Minister (OPDM) (2006) *Buildings Regulations Part M Amendment 2003*. RIBA Bookshop, London.

Sangster K (1997) *Costing Lifetime Homes*. Joseph Rowntree Foundation, York.

Seelman K (2001) Science and technology policy: is disability a missing factor? In: Albrecht GL, Seelman KD, Bury M (eds) (2001) *Handbook of Disability Studies*. Sage Publications, California.

World Health Organization (2002) *Towards a Common Language for Functioning, Disability and Health. The International Classification of Functioning, Disability and Health*. Available at: www.who.int/classification/icf.

# Appendices

# APPENDIX I Further reading

## Acts, statutory instruments and official publications

### European Union

### Ireland

Building Control Act 1990

Building Control Regulations 1997, SI 496 of 1997

Building Regulations (Amendment) Regulations 2000, SI 179 of 2000

Code of Practice for the Management of Fire Safety in Places of Assembly 1989

Employment Equality Act 1998

Equal Status Act 2000

Fire Services Act 1981

National Development Plan 1999

Safety, Health and Welfare at Work Act 1989

Safety, Health and Welfare at Work (Signs) Regulations 1995, SI 132 of 1995

Technical Guidance Documents to the Building Regulations 2000, especially those to Part K, Stairways, ramps and guards, and Part M, Access and facilities for disabled persons

### United Kingdom

COM (2000) 284 final, May 2000: Communication from the Commission to the Council, the European Parliament, the Economic and Social Committee and the Commission of the Regions: Towards a barrier-free Europe for people with disabilities

Council decision (2000/750/EC), November 2000: Council decision establishing a community action programme to combat discrimination (2001–2006)

## Standards and codes of practice

BS 4467: 1991: Anthropometric and ergonomic recommendations for dimensions in designing for the elderly

BS 5378: Part 1: 1980: Safety signs and colours. Part 1: Specification for colour and design

BS 5499: 1990: Fire safety signs, notices and graphic symbols

BS 5588: Part 8: 1999: Fire precautions in the design and construction of buildings: means of escape for disabled people

BS 5655: 1986: Lifts and service lifts

BS 5776: 1996: Specification for powered stair lifts

BS 5810: 1979: Code of practice for access for the disabled to buildings

BS 5839: Part 1: 1988: Code of practice for system design, installation and servicing

BS 5887: 1980: Specification for mobile, manually operated patient lifting devices

BS 5900: 1991: Specification for powered domestic home lifts

BS 6034: 1990: Specification for public information symbols

BS 6083: Part 4: 1981: Specification for magnetic field strength in audio-frequency induction loops for hearing aid purposes

BS 6130: 1993: Code of practice for powered lifting platforms for use by people with disabilities

BS 6206: 1981: Specification for impact performance requirements for flat safety glass and safety plastics for use in buildings

BS 6259: 1982: Code of practice for planning and installation of sound systems

BS 6262: 1982: Code of practice for glazing for buildings

BS 6418: 1989: Specification for cordless audio transmission devices using infra-red radiation

BS 6440: 1983: Code of practice for powered lifting platforms for use by disabled persons

BS 7036: Code of practice for safety at powered doors for pedestrian use

BS 7443: 1991: Specification for sound systems for emergency purposes

BS 7594: 1993: Code of practice for audible frequency induction loop systems

BS 8300: 2001: Design of buildings to meet the needs of disabled people

## Periodicals

*Access by Design* (quarterly)
Centre for Accessible Environments, Nutmeg House, 60 Gainsford
Street, London SEI 2NY, England. Fax: 0044 207 357 8183, email:
info@cae.org.uk
*Crisp and Clear – European Magazine on Design for All* (irregular)
Danish Centre for Accessibility, Graham Bells Vej 1A, DK-8200 Aarhus
N, Denmark. Fax: 00 45 86 78 37 30
*Design Insight – Journal of the JMU Access Partnership* (quarterly)
JMU, 105 Judd Street, London WC1 9NE, England.
Fax: 00 44 207 387 7109, email: publications@jmuaccess.org.uk
*European Institute for Design and Disability Journal* (quarterly)
Institut TLP, Post Box 1186, 56831 Traben-Trarbach, Germany.
Fax: 00 49 6541 9237

## Other publications

Access Committee for England (1996) *Designing Housing for Successive
Generations*. Access Committee for England, London.
Ambrose I (1996) *Elimination of Architectural Barriers: accessibility in
public buildings*. Danish Building Research Institute, Denmark.
Arts Council of Northern Ireland (1999) *Arts and Disability Handbook*.
Arts Council of Northern Ireland, Belfast.
Asthma Society of Ireland (1994) *Dust in the Home*. Asthma Society of
Ireland, Dublin.
Australian Building Codes Board (1996) *Building Code of Australia Access
Provisions Review*. Australian Building Codes Board, Canberra,
Australia.
Barker P, Fraser J (2001) *Sign Design Guide – a guide to inclusive signage*.
JMU and Sign Design Society, London.
Barker P, Barrick J, Wilson R (1997) *Building Sight: a handbook of building
and interior design solutions to include the needs of visually impaired
people*. HMSO in association with RNIB, London.
Bone S (1996) *Buildings for All to Use*. CIRIA, London.
Brewerton J, Darton D (eds) (1997) *Designing Lifetime Homes*. Joseph
Rowntree Foundation, York.
Carroll C, Cowans J, Darton D (1999) *Meeting Part M and Designing
Lifetime Homes*. Joseph Rowntree Foundation, York.
Centre for Accessible Environments (1999) *Access to ATMs: UK design
guidelines*. Centre for Accessible Environments, London.
Cobbold C (1997) *A Cost-Benefit Analysis of Lifetime Homes*. Joseph
Rowntree Foundation, York.

Department of the Environment, Transport and the Regions (1999) *Accessible Thresholds in New Housing: guidance for house builders and designers*. Department of the Environment, Transport and the Regions, London.

Dublin Diocesan Jubilee Committee (2000) *It's My Church Too: the inclusion of people with disability in the life of the church*. Dublin Diocesan Jubilee Committee, Dublin.

English Heritage (1999) *Easy Access to Historic Properties*. English Heritage, London.

Fieldfare Trust (1997) *BT Countryside for All: a good practice guide to disabled people's access in the countryside*. Fieldfare Trust, Sheffield.

Football Stadia Advisory Design Council (1992) *Designing for Spectators with Disabilities*. Football Stadia Advisory Design Council, London.

Forestry Commission (1998) *A Guide to Easy Access: a national gazeteer*. Forestry Commission, Edinburgh.

Foster L (1997) *Access to the Historic Environment: meeting the needs of disabled people*. RNIB, London.

Frontend (2000) *Accessibility and Usability for e-Government: a primer for public sector officials*. Frontend, Dublin.

Gill J (2000) *Which Button? Designing user interfaces for people with visual impairments*. RNIB, London.

Gleeson B (1999) *Geographies of Disability*. Routledge, London.

Goldsmith S (1997) *Designing for the Disabled: a new paradigm*. Architectural Press, London.

Goldsmith S (2000) *Universal Design*. RIBA, London.

Heritage Council (1999) *Forestry and the Natural Heritage*. Heritage Council, Kilkenny, Ireland.

Heritage Council (2000) *Heritage Awareness in Ireland*. Heritage Council, Kilkenny, Ireland.

Hickie D (1997) *Evaluation of Environmental Designations in Ireland*. Heritage Council, Kilkenny, Ireland.

HMSO (1997) *Safety at Street Works and Roads Works*. HMSO, London.

Hodge SJ (1995) *Creating and Managing Woodlands Around Towns*. Forestry Commission Handbook 11. Forestry Commission, HMSO, London.

Holmes-Siedle J (1996) *Barrier-Free Design: a manual for building designers and managers*. Butterworth Architecture, London.

Human Rights and Equal Opportunity Commission (1997) *Advisory Notes on Access to Premises*. Human Rights and Equal Opportunity Commission, Sydney, Australia.

Imrie R (1996) *Disability and the City: international perspectives*. Sage Publications, London.

Imrie R, Hall P (2001) *Inclusive Design: designing and developing accessible environments*. Taylor and Francis, London.

McGeer P, Fidderman H (2000) *Fit for the Job: health, safety and disability at work*. Eclipse Group, London.

Museums and Galleries Commission (1994) *Disability Resource Directory for Museums*. Museums and Galleries Commission, London.

Museums and Galleries Commission (1997) *Access to Museums and Galleries for People with Disabilities*. Museums and Galleries Commission, London.

National Rehabilitation Board (1999) Submission to the Department of the Environment and Local Government on its consultation document, Revision of Part M: Building Regulations. Proposals for making new dwellings visitable by people with disabilities. National Rehabilitation Board, Dublin.

Northern Officer Group (1993) *Personal Emergency Egress Plans*. Northern Officer Group, Centre for Accessible Environments (CAE), London.

Office for Official Publications of the European Communities (1999) *Making Workplaces Accessible: a guide to integration*. Office for Official Publications of the European Communities, Luxembourg.

Office of the Rail Regulator (2000) *Train and Station Services for Disabled Passengers*. Office of the Rail Regulator, London.

Penton J (2001) *Widening the Eye of the Needle: access to church buildings for people with disabilities*. Church House Publishing, London.

Pickles J, Taylor D (1999) *Housing for Varying Needs: a design guide – Part M: houses and flats*. HMSO, London.

RNIB (1999) *New European Standards on Man-Machine Interface for Card Systems*. RNIB, London.

RNIB Scientific Research Unit (2000) *Tiresias – a family of typefaces designed for legibility on screens, signs and labels*. RNIB Scientific Research Unit, London.

Shields TJ (1993) *Fire and Disabled People in Buildings, BR 231*. BRE, Watford.

Shields TJ, Dunlop KE, Silcock GWH (1996) *Escape of Disabled People from Fire: a measurement and classification capability for assessing fire risk, BR301*. BRE, London.

Stoneham J, Thoday P (1996) *Landscape Design for Elderly and Disabled People*. Garden Art Press, Suffolk.

The following are all published by the Centre for Accessible Environments, Nutmeg House, 60 Gainsford Street, London SE1 2NY, England. Fax 00 44 207 357 8183, email: info@cae.org.uk

Fearns D (1999) *Access Audits: a guide and checklists for appraising the accessibility of buildings for disabled users*.

Palfreyman T (1994) *Designing for Accessibility: an introductory guide*.

Thorpe S (1994) *Reading and Using Plans: specifiers' handbooks*:

1. Electrical Controls
2. Wheelchair Stair Lifts and Platform Lifts
3. Automatic Door Controls
4. Internal Floor Finishes: improving access for all.

Thorpe S (1995) *House Adaptations*.
Thorpe S (1998) *Good Loo Design Guide: advice on WC provision for disabled people in public buildings*.

# APPENDIX II  A comparison anthropometric table across gender and age groups

The Ergonomics Society (www.ergonomics.org.uk) is a charitable organisation based in the UK.

It provides the following website www.ergonomics4schools.com to encourage learning about ergonomics.

The anthropometric tables used here have been sourced from this site.

| 1. Stature | 1st %-le | 5th%-le | 50th %-le | 95th%-le | 99th%-le | SD |
|---|---|---|---|---|---|---|
| | | | | | | |
| men aged 19 to 65 years | 1575 | 1625 | 1740 | 1855 | 1900 | 70 |
| women aged 19 to 65 years | 1465 | 1505 | 1610 | 1710 | 1750 | 62 |
| male students | 1625 | 1670 | 1770 | 1875 | 1915 | 62 |
| female students | 1500 | 1545 | 1650 | 1755 | 1795 | 63 |
| elderly men 65 years and above | 1460 | 1515 | 1640 | 1770 | 1820 | 77 |
| elderly women 65 years and above | 1350 | 1400 | 1515 | 1630 | 1680 | 70 |
| men aged 19 to 65 years | 1575 | 1625 | 1740 | 1855 | 1900 | 70 |
| women aged 19 to 65 years | 1465 | 1505 | 1610 | 1710 | 1750 | 62 |
| male students | 1625 | 1670 | 1770 | 1875 | 1915 | 62 |
| boys 3–4 year olds | | 930 | 1020 | 1110 | | 56 |
| boys 5–7 year olds | | 1045 | 1170 | 1295 | | 74 |
| boys 8–11 year olds | | 1220 | 1360 | 1495 | | 85 |
| boys 12–14 year olds | | 1385 | 1555 | 1725 | | 104 |
| boys 15–18 year olds | | 1610 | 1735 | 1855 | | 75 |
| girls 3–4 year olds | | 905 | 1010 | 1115 | | 63 |
| girls 5–7 year olds | | 1040 | 1160 | 1280 | | 74 |
| girls 8–11 year olds | | 1210 | 1360 | 1510 | | 92 |
| girls 12–14 year olds | | 1410 | 1545 | 1680 | | 82 |
| girls 15–18 year olds | | 1520 | 1620 | 1715 | | 60 |

| 2. Eye height | 1st %-le | 5th%-le | 50th %-le | 95th%-le | 99th%-le | SD |
|---|---|---|---|---|---|---|
| men aged 19 to 65 years | 1460 | 1510 | 1625 | 1745 | 1790 | 71 |
| women aged 19 to 65 years | 1345 | 1390 | 1490 | 1595 | 1640 | 63 |
| male students | 1510 | 1555 | 1660 | 1760 | 1805 | 63 |
| female students | 1380 | 1425 | 1530 | 1635 | 1680 | 64 |
| elderly men 65 years and above | 1355 | 1405 | 1535 | 1665 | 1720 | 78 |
| elderly women 65 years and above | 1240 | 1285 | 1405 | 1520 | 1570 | 71 |
| boys 3–4 year olds | | 825 | 915 | 1005 | | 54 |
| boys 5–7 year olds | | 930 | 1055 | 1175 | | 75 |
| boys 8–11 year olds | | 1070 | 1215 | 1360 | | 88 |
| boys 12–14 year olds | | 1270 | 1440 | 1610 | | 103 |
| boys 15–18 year olds | | 1490 | 1615 | 1740 | | 76 |
| girls 3–4 year olds | | 800 | 910 | 1020 | | 68 |
| girls 5–7 year olds | | 915 | 1045 | 1180 | | 81 |
| girls 8–11 year olds | | 1095 | 1245 | 1395 | | 92 |
| girls 12–14 year olds | | 1295 | 1430 | 1565 | | 82 |
| girls 15–18 year olds | | 1410 | 1510 | 1610 | | 60 |

| 3. Cervical height | 1st %-le | 5th%-le | 50th %-le | 95th%-le | 99th%-le | SD |
|---|---|---|---|---|---|---|
| men aged 19 to 65 years | 1330 | 1375 | 1485 | 1595 | 1640 | 67 |
| women aged 19 to 65 years | 1240 | 1280 | 1375 | 1470 | 1510 | 59 |
| male students | 1375 | 1415 | 1515 | 1610 | 1650 | 59 |
| female students | 1270 | 1310 | 1410 | 1510 | 1550 | 60 |
| elderly men 65 years and above | 1235 | 1285 | 1405 | 1525 | 1575 | 73 |
| elderly women 65 years and above | 1140 | 1185 | 1295 | 1405 | 1450 | 67 |

| 4. Shoulder height | 1st %-le | 5th%-le | 50th %-le | 95th%-le | 99th%-le | SD |
|---|---|---|---|---|---|---|
| men aged 19 to 65 years | 1265 | 1310 | 1415 | 1525 | 1570 | 65 |
| women aged 19 to 65 years | 1165 | 1210 | 1310 | 1410 | 1455 | 62 |
| male students | 1310 | 1350 | 1445 | 1540 | 1580 | 58 |
| female students | 1200 | 1240 | 1345 | 1445 | 1490 | 62 |
| elderly men 65 years and above | 1170 | 1220 | 1335 | 1455 | 1505 | 72 |
| elderly women 65 years and above | 1070 | 1120 | 1235 | 1345 | 1395 | 69 |
| boys 3–4 year olds | | 735 | 805 | 870 | | 42 |
| boys 5–7 year olds | | 820 | 925 | 1025 | | 62 |
| boys 8–11 year olds | | 960 | 1090 | 1220 | | 79 |
| boys 12–14 year olds | | 1120 | 1270 | 1425 | | 92 |
| boys 15–18 year olds | | 1310 | 1420 | 1530 | | 67 |
| girls 3–4 year olds | | 700 | 795 | 885 | | 56 |
| girls 5–7 year olds | | 805 | 910 | 1020 | | 64 |
| girls 8–11 year olds | | 950 | 1090 | 1230 | | 85 |
| girls 12–14 year olds | | 1130 | 1255 | 1380 | | 75 |
| girls 15–18 year olds | | 1225 | 1315 | 1405 | | 54 |

| 5. Elbow height | 1st %-le | 5th%-le | 50th %-le | 95th%-le | 99th%-le | SD |
|---|---|---|---|---|---|---|
| men aged 19 to 65 years | 960 | 995 | 1080 | 1165 | 1200 | 52 |
| women aged 19 to 65 years | 875 | 905 | 980 | 1060 | 1090 | 47 |
| male students | 995 | 1025 | 1100 | 1175 | 1210 | 46 |
| female students | 895 | 930 | 1010 | 1085 | 1120 | 48 |
| elderly men 65 years and above | 890 | 925 | 1020 | 1115 | 1155 | 57 |
| elderly women 65 years and above | 800 | 835 | 925 | 1010 | 1050 | 53 |
| boys 3–4 year olds | | 550 | 615 | 680 | | 40 |
| boys 5–7 year olds | | 620 | 705 | 790 | | 51 |
| boys 8–11 year olds | | 730 | 840 | 945 | | 66 |
| boys 12–14 year olds | | 860 | 970 | 1085 | | 68 |
| boys 15–18 year olds | | 995 | 1080 | 1170 | | 53 |
| girls 3–4 year olds | | 530 | 605 | 680 | | 45 |
| girls 5–7 year olds | | 610 | 695 | 780 | | 52 |
| girls 8–11 year olds | | 720 | 835 | 950 | | 69 |
| girls 12–14 year olds | | 865 | 965 | 1065 | | 60 |
| girls 15–18 year olds | | 930 | 1005 | 1080 | | 45 |

| 6. Hip height | 1st %le | 5th%-le | 50th %-le | 95th%-le | 99th%-le | SD |
|---|---|---|---|---|---|---|
| men aged 19 to 65 years | 800 | 830 | 910 | 995 | 1025 | 49 |
| women aged 19 to 65 years | 715 | 745 | 815 | 885 | 915 | 42 |
| male students | 830 | 860 | 930 | 1000 | 1030 | 43 |
| female students | 735 | 765 | 835 | 905 | 935 | 43 |
| elderly men 65 years and above | 735 | 775 | 860 | 950 | 985 | 54 |
| elderly women 65 years and above | 655 | 690 | 765 | 845 | 880 | 48 |
| boys 3–4 year olds | | 415 | 480 | 545 | | 39 |
| boys 5–7 year olds | | 505 | 595 | 680 | | 53 |
| boys 8–11 year olds | | 620 | 715 | 810 | | 57 |
| boys 12–14 year olds | | 740 | 835 | 935 | | 59 |
| boys 15–18 year olds | | 835 | 915 | 995 | | 49 |
| girls 3–4 year olds | | 415 | 485 | 550 | | 41 |
| girls 5–7 year olds | | 505 | 575 | 650 | | 45 |
| girls 8–11 year olds | | 605 | 705 | 805 | | 60 |
| girls 12–14 year olds | | 715 | 800 | 880 | | 49 |
| girls 15–18 year olds | | 750 | 820 | 885 | | 40 |

| 7. Knuckle height | 1st %le | 5th%-le | 50th %-le | 95th%-le | 99th%-le | SD |
|---|---|---|---|---|---|---|
| men aged 19 to 65 years | 665 | 695 | 765 | 835 | 860 | 42 |
| women aged 19 to 65 years | 615 | 640 | 700 | 760 | 785 | 37 |
| male students | 690 | 715 | 775 | 840 | 865 | 38 |
| female students | 630 | 655 | 715 | 780 | 805 | 38 |
| elderly men 65 years and above | 610 | 645 | 720 | 795 | 830 | 47 |
| elderly women 65 years and above | 560 | 590 | 660 | 725 | 755 | 42 |
| boys 3–4 year olds | | 375 | 425 | 470 | | 29 |
| boys 5–7 year olds | | 420 | 480 | 545 | | 38 |
| boys 8–11 year olds | | 500 | 580 | 655 | | 47 |
| boys 12–14 year olds | | 595 | 670 | 750 | | 48 |
| boys 15–18 year olds | | 675 | 745 | 815 | | 43 |
| girls 3–4 year olds | | 370 | 430 | 485 | | 36 |
| girls 5–7 year olds | | 420 | 495 | 565 | | 43 |
| girls 8–11 year olds | | 520 | 600 | 685 | | 50 |
| girls 12–14 year olds | | 605 | 680 | 760 | | 46 |
| girls 15–18 year olds | | 665 | 720 | 780 | | 35 |

| 8. Fingertip height | 1st %-le | 5th%-le | 50th %-le | 95th%-le | 99th%-le | SD |
|---|---|---|---|---|---|---|
| men aged 19 to 65 years | 555 | 580 | 640 | 705 | 730 | 38 |
| women aged 19 to 65 years | 515 | 540 | 595 | 650 | 670 | 34 |
| male students | 575 | 600 | 655 | 710 | 730 | 34 |
| female students | 530 | 550 | 610 | 665 | 690 | 34 |
| elderly men 65 years and above | 510 | 535 | 605 | 675 | 700 | 42 |
| elderly women 65 years and above | 470 | 495 | 560 | 620 | 645 | 38 |
| boys 3–4 year olds | | 305 | 350 | 395 | | 28 |
| boys 5–7 year olds | | 335 | 395 | 460 | | 37 |
| boys 8–11 year olds | | 410 | 485 | 555 | | 44 |
| boys 12–14 year olds | | 485 | 560 | 635 | | 46 |
| boys 15–18 year olds | | 555 | 625 | 695 | | 43 |
| girls 3–4 year olds | | 295 | 355 | 410 | | 34 |
| girls 5–7 year olds | | 345 | 410 | 480 | | 41 |
| girls 8–11 year olds | | 425 | 505 | 585 | | 48 |
| girls 12–14 year olds | | 495 | 570 | 650 | | 46 |
| girls 15–18 year olds | | 550 | 610 | 665 | | 35 |

| 9. Sitting height | 1st %-le | 5th%-le | 50th %-le | 95th%-le | 99th%-le | SD |
|---|---|---|---|---|---|---|
| men aged 19 to 65 years | 825 | 850 | 910 | 970 | 995 | 37 |
| women aged 19 to 65 years | 765 | 790 | 845 | 900 | 925 | 34 |
| male students | 850 | 875 | 925 | 980 | 1000 | 32 |
| female students | 785 | 810 | 865 | 925 | 950 | 35 |
| elderly men 65 years and above | 730 | 760 | 830 | 895 | 925 | 42 |
| elderly women 65 years and above | 650 | 685 | 770 | 855 | 890 | 51 |
| boys 3–4 year olds | | 535 | 585 | 630 | | 28 |
| boys 5–7 year olds | | 585 | 640 | 700 | | 35 |
| boys 8–11 year olds | | 645 | 710 | 775 | | 39 |
| boys 12–14 year olds | | 705 | 795 | 885 | | 55 |
| boys 15–18 year olds | | 825 | 900 | 970 | | 44 |
| girls 3–4 year olds | | 520 | 575 | 625 | | 32 |
| girls 5–7 year olds | | 575 | 635 | 695 | | 37 |
| girls 8–11 year olds | | 645 | 715 | 780 | | 42 |
| girls 12–14 year olds | | 725 | 805 | 880 | | 47 |
| girls 15–18 year olds | | 800 | 855 | 905 | | 33 |

| 10. Sitting eye height | 1st %-le | 5th%-le | 50th %-le | 95th%-le | 99th%-le | SD |
|---|---|---|---|---|---|---|
| men aged 19 to 65 years | 710 | 740 | 800 | 860 | 885 | 38 |
| women aged 19 to 65 years | 665 | 685 | 740 | 790 | 810 | 32 |
| male students | 735 | 760 | 815 | 870 | 890 | 33 |
| female students | 680 | 705 | 755 | 810 | 830 | 32 |
| elderly men 65 years and above | 625 | 655 | 730 | 800 | 830 | 43 |
| elderly women 65 years and above | 565 | 595 | 675 | 750 | 780 | 47 |
| boys 3–4 year olds | | 430 | 475 | 520 | | 28 |
| boys 5–7 year olds | | 470 | 525 | 585 | | 35 |
| boys 8–11 year olds | | 535 | 595 | 650 | | 36 |
| boys 12–14 year olds | | 595 | 685 | 770 | | 53 |
| boys 15–18 year olds | | 715 | 785 | 850 | | 41 |
| girls 3–4 year olds | | 405 | 465 | 520 | | 35 |
| girls 5–7 year olds | | 465 | 525 | 590 | | 39 |
| girls 8–11 year olds | | 540 | 605 | 675 | | 41 |
| girls 12–14 year olds | | 620 | 695 | 765 | | 45 |
| girls 15–18 year olds | | 690 | 740 | 790 | | 31 |

| 11. Sitting shoulder height | 1st %-le | 5th%-le | 50th %-le | 95th%-le | 99th%-le | SD |
|---|---|---|---|---|---|---|
| men aged 19 to 65 years | 520 | 545 | 600 | 655 | 680 | 34 |
| women aged 19 to 65 years | 490 | 510 | 565 | 615 | 640 | 32 |
| male students | 540 | 560 | 610 | 660 | 680 | 31 |
| female students | 505 | 525 | 580 | 630 | 655 | 32 |
| elderly men 65 years and above | 450 | 480 | 545 | 610 | 640 | 40 |
| elderly women 65 years and above | 405 | 435 | 515 | 590 | 625 | 47 |
| boys 3–4 year olds | | 315 | 355 | 395 | | 24 |
| boys 5–7 year olds | | 345 | 390 | 440 | | 29 |
| boys 8–11 year olds | | 395 | 450 | 500 | | 32 |
| boys 12–14 year olds | | 445 | 510 | 580 | | 40 |
| boys 15–18 year olds | | 520 | 580 | 635 | | 35 |
| girls 3–4 year olds | | 315 | 355 | 395 | | 24 |
| girls 5–7 year olds | | 345 | 390 | 440 | | 29 |
| girls 8–11 year olds | | 395 | 450 | 500 | | 32 |
| girls 12–14 year olds | | 445 | 510 | 580 | | 40 |
| girls 15–18 year olds | | 520 | 580 | 635 | | 35 |

| 12. Elbow rest height | 1st %-le | 5th%-le | 50th %-le | 95th%-le | 99th%-le | SD |
|---|---|---|---|---|---|---|
| men aged 19 to 65 years | 175 | 190 | 240 | 285 | 305 | 28 |
| women aged 19 to 65 years | 170 | 185 | 225 | 265 | 285 | 24 |
| male students | 185 | 200 | 245 | 285 | 300 | 25 |
| female students | 175 | 190 | 235 | 275 | 290 | 24 |
| elderly men 65 years and above | 140 | 160 | 210 | 250 | 280 | 31 |
| elderly women 65 years and above | 115 | 140 | 195 | 250 | 275 | 35 |
| boys 3–4 year olds | | 120 | 155 | 190 | | 21 |
| boys 5–7 year olds | | 135 | 170 | 205 | | 23 |
| boys 8–11 year olds | | 150 | 190 | 230 | | 24 |
| boys 12–14 year olds | | 165 | 210 | 255 | | 29 |
| boys 15–18 year olds | | 185 | 235 | 285 | | 30 |
| girls 3–4 year olds | | 115 | 145 | 175 | | 19 |
| girls 5–7 year olds | | 130 | 160 | 195 | | 21 |
| girls 8–11 year olds | | 145 | 185 | 230 | | 26 |
| girls 12–14 year olds | | 155 | 210 | 265 | | 33 |
| girls 15–18 year olds | | 185 | 230 | 270 | | 26 |

| 13. Thigh clearance | 1st %-le | 5th%-le | 50th %-le | 95th%-le | 99th%-le | SD |
|---|---|---|---|---|---|---|
| men aged 19 to 65 years | 115 | 125 | 150 | 175 | 190 | 16 |
| women aged 19 to 65 years | 90 | 105 | 140 | 170 | 185 | 21 |
| male students | 120 | 130 | 155 | 175 | 185 | 14 |
| female students | 95 | 110 | 140 | 175 | 190 | 21 |
| elderly men 65 years and above | 90 | 105 | 135 | 160 | 175 | 18 |
| elderly women 65 years and above | 90 | 105 | 140 | 175 | 190 | 22 |
| boys 3–4 year olds | | 70 | 90 | 105 | | 12 |
| boys 5–7 year olds | | 75 | 95 | 120 | | 14 |
| boys 8–11 year olds | | 95 | 115 | 140 | | 14 |
| boys 12–14 year olds | | 105 | 130 | 160 | | 16 |
| boys 15–18 year olds | | 125 | 150 | 180 | | 17 |
| girls 3–4 year olds | | 60 | 85 | 105 | | 13 |
| girls 5–7 year olds | | 75 | 95 | 120 | | 14 |
| girls 8–11 year olds | | 90 | 120 | 145 | | 16 |
| girls 12–14 year olds | | 110 | 135 | 160 | | 16 |
| girls 15–18 year olds | | 120 | 145 | 170 | | 15 |

| 14. Standard seat height | 1st %-le | 5th%-le | 50th %-le | 95th%-le | 99th%-le | SD |
|---|---|---|---|---|---|---|
| men aged 19 to 65 years | 350 | 365 | 415 | 460 | 480 | 28 |
| women aged 19 to 65 years | 325 | 340 | 380 | 420 | 435 | 24 |
| male students | 365 | 380 | 420 | 460 | 480 | 25 |
| female students | 335 | 350 | 390 | 430 | 445 | 24 |
| elderly men 65 years and above | 320 | 340 | 390 | 440 | 460 | 31 |
| elderly women 65 years and above | 295 | 315 | 355 | 400 | 420 | 27 |

| 15. Knee height | 1st %-le | 5th%-le | 50th %-le | 95th%-le | 99th%-le | SD |
|---|---|---|---|---|---|---|
| men aged 19 to 65 years | 475 | 495 | 540 | 590 | 610 | 29 |
| women aged 19 to 65 years | 440 | 455 | 495 | 535 | 555 | 24 |
| male students | 495 | 510 | 555 | 595 | 610 | 25 |
| female students | 450 | 470 | 510 | 550 | 565 | 25 |
| elderly men 65 years and above | 445 | 465 | 515 | 570 | 590 | 33 |
| elderly women 65 years and above | 390 | 410 | 465 | 520 | 540 | 33 |
| boys 3–4 year olds | | 265 | 300 | 335 | | 22 |
| boys 5–7 year olds | | 310 | 360 | 410 | | 30 |
| boys 8–11 year olds | | 375 | 430 | 485 | | 34 |
| boys 12–14 year olds | | 440 | 500 | 560 | | 37 |
| boys 15–18 year olds | | 500 | 545 | 590 | | 28 |
| girls 3–4 year olds | | 255 | 300 | 340 | | 25 |
| girls 5–7 year olds | | 305 | 355 | 400 | | 28 |
| girls 8–11 year olds | | 370 | 430 | 485 | | 35 |
| girls 12–14 year olds | | 435 | 485 | 530 | | 30 |
| girls 15–18 year olds | | 455 | 500 | 540 | | 26 |

| 16. Popliteal height | 1st %-le | 5th%-le | 50th %-le | 95th%-le | 99th%-le | SD |
|---|---|---|---|---|---|---|
| men aged 19 to 65 years | 385 | 400 | 440 | 480 | 500 | 25 |
| women aged 19 to 65 years | 365 | 380 | 415 | 450 | 465 | 21 |
| male students | 400 | 415 | 450 | 485 | 500 | 22 |
| female students | 375 | 390 | 425 | 460 | 475 | 21 |
| elderly men 65 years and above | 360 | 375 | 420 | 465 | 485 | 28 |
| elderly women 65 years and above | 320 | 340 | 385 | 435 | 455 | 29 |
| boys 3–4 year olds | | 205 | 245 | 280 | | 21 |
| boys 5–7 year olds | | 250 | 295 | 340 | | 27 |
| boys 8–11 year olds | | 300 | 350 | 400 | | 29 |
| boys 12–14 year olds | | 355 | 405 | 455 | | 31 |
| boys 15–18 year olds | | 395 | 440 | 485 | | 27 |
| girls 3–4 year olds | | 210 | 245 | 275 | | 20 |
| girls 5–7 year olds | | 250 | 290 | 330 | | 24 |
| girls 8–11 year olds | | 305 | 355 | 400 | | 30 |
| girls 12–14 year olds | | 350 | 390 | 430 | | 25 |
| girls 15–18 year olds | | 360 | 405 | 445 | | 25 |

| 17. Buttock knee length | 1st %-le | 5th%-le | 50th %-le | 95th%-le | 99th%-le | SD |
|---|---|---|---|---|---|---|
| men aged 19 to 65 years | 520 | 540 | 595 | 645 | 665 | 31 |
| women aged 19 to 65 years | 500 | 520 | 570 | 620 | 640 | 30 |
| male students | 540 | 560 | 605 | 650 | 665 | 27 |
| female students | 515 | 535 | 585 | 635 | 655 | 30 |
| elderly men 65 years and above | 485 | 510 | 565 | 620 | 645 | 35 |
| elderly women 65 years and above | 485 | 510 | 560 | 615 | 635 | 32 |
| boys 3–4 year olds | | 275 | 315 | 350 | 23 | |
| boys 5–7 year olds | | 320 | 370 | 420 | 31 | |
| boys 8–11 year olds | | 390 | 450 | 510 | 36 | |
| boys 12–14 year olds | | 460 | 525 | 590 | 39 | |
| boys 15–18 year olds | | 530 | 580 | 630 | 30 | |
| girls 3–4 year olds | | 275 | 320 | 360 | 25 | |
| girls 5–7 year olds | | 320 | 375 | 425 | 32 | |
| girls 8–11 year olds | | 390 | 455 | 525 | 41 | |
| girls 12–14 year olds | | 470 | 530 | 585 | 35 | |
| girls 15–18 year olds | | 510 | 555 | 600 | 28 | |

| 18. Buttock popliteal length | 1st %-le | 5th%-le | 50th %-le | 95th%-le | 99th%-le | SD |
|---|---|---|---|---|---|---|
| men aged 19 to 65 years | 420 | 440 | 495 | 550 | 570 | 33 |
| women aged 19 to 65 years | 410 | 430 | 480 | 535 | 555 | 31 |
| male students | 440 | 455 | 505 | 550 | 570 | 29 |
| female students | 425 | 445 | 495 | 545 | 565 | 31 |
| elderly men 65 years and above | 410 | 430 | 485 | 540 | 560 | 32 |
| elderly women 65 years and above | 400 | 420 | 475 | 530 | 550 | 32 |
| boys 3–4 year olds | | 230 | 260 | 285 | | 18 |
| boys 5–7 year olds | | 255 | 305 | 350 | | 29 |
| boys 8–11 year olds | | 315 | 370 | 425 | | 33 |
| boys 12–14 year olds | | 380 | 435 | 495 | | 36 |
| boys 15–18 year olds | | 440 | 490 | 545 | | 32 |
| girls 3–4 year olds | | 230 | 270 | 305 | | 23 |
| girls 5–7 year olds | | 270 | 315 | 360 | | 28 |
| girls 8–11 year olds | | 330 | 385 | 445 | | 35 |
| girls 12–14 year olds | | 395 | 445 | 495 | | 30 |
| girls 15–18 year olds | | 435 | 480 | 520 | | 26 |

| 19. Shoulder breadth (bideltoid) | 1st %-le | 5th%-le | 50th %-le | 95th%-le | 99th%-le | SD |
|---|---|---|---|---|---|---|
| men aged 19 to 65 years | 395 | 415 | 460 | 500 | 520 | 27 |
| women aged 19 to 65 years | 355 | 370 | 415 | 460 | 475 | 26 |
| male students | 415 | 430 | 470 | 505 | 520 | 23 |
| female students | 365 | 380 | 425 | 470 | 485 | 27 |
| elderly men 65 years and above | 360 | 375 | 420 | 460 | 475 | 25 |
| elderly women 65 years and above | 320 | 335 | 375 | 410 | 430 | 23 |
| boys 3–4 year olds | | 235 | 260 | 285 | | 16 |
| boys 5–7 year olds | | 250 | 285 | 325 | | 23 |
| boys 8–11 year olds | | 280 | 330 | 375 | | 28 |
| boys 12–14 year olds | | 320 | 375 | 430 | | 32 |
| boys 15–18 year olds | | 385 | 435 | 490 | | 32 |
| girls 3–4 year olds | | 230 | 260 | 285 | | 17 |
| girls 5–7 year olds | | 245 | 285 | 320 | | 23 |
| girls 8–11 year olds | | 275 | 325 | 375 | | 30 |
| girls 12–14 year olds | | 320 | 370 | 420 | | 29 |
| girls 15–18 year olds | | 360 | 395 | 430 | | 22 |

| 20. Biacromial breadth | 1st %-le | 5th%-le | 50th %-le | 95th%-le | 99th%-le | SD |
|---|---|---|---|---|---|---|
| men aged 19 to 65 years | 350 | 365 | 400 | 440 | 455 | 22 |
| women aged 19 to 65 years | 315 | 325 | 355 | 385 | 395 | 18 |
| male students | 365 | 375 | 410 | 440 | 455 | 20 |
| female students | 320 | 335 | 365 | 390 | 405 | 18 |
| elderly men 65 years and above | 315 | 330 | 365 | 400 | 415 | 21 |
| elderly women 65 years and above | 280 | 290 | 320 | 345 | 350 | 15 |
| boys 3–4 year olds | | 205 | 230 | 255 | | 14 |
| boys 5–7 year olds | | 230 | 265 | 295 | | 19 |
| boys 8–11 year olds | | 265 | 300 | 335 | | 20 |
| boys 12–14 year olds | | 295 | 340 | 380 | | 26 |
| boys 15–18 year olds | | 345 | 385 | 420 | | 23 |
| girls 3–4 year olds | | 205 | 235 | 260 | | 15 |
| girls 5–7 year olds | | 235 | 260 | 285 | | 16 |
| girls 8–11 year olds | | 260 | 300 | 335 | | 23 |
| girls 12–14 year olds | | 300 | 335 | 370 | | 22 |
| girls 15–18 year olds | | 330 | 355 | 385 | | 17 |

| 21. Elbow to elbow breadth | 1st %-le | 5th%-le | 50th %-le | 95th%-le | 99th%-le | SD |
|---|---|---|---|---|---|---|
| men aged 19 to 65 years | 370 | 390 | 450 | 510 | 535 | 35 |
| women aged 19 to 65 years | 260 | 300 | 385 | 475 | 510 | 54 |
| male students | 385 | 405 | 460 | 510 | 530 | 31 |
| female students | 270 | 305 | 395 | 485 | 520 | 54 |
| elderly men 65 years and above | 400 | 430 | 500 | 570 | 595 | 42 |
| elderly women 65 years and above | 350 | 380 | 455 | 530 | 560 | 46 |

| 22. Hip breadth | 1st %-le | 5th%-le | 50th %-le | 95th%-le | 99th%-le | SD |
|---|---|---|---|---|---|---|
| men aged 19 to 65 years | 300 | 315 | 360 | 400 | 415 | 25 |
| women aged 19 to 65 years | 295 | 320 | 375 | 430 | 450 | 34 |
| male students | 315 | 330 | 365 | 400 | 415 | 22 |
| female students | 305 | 325 | 385 | 440 | 460 | 34 |
| elderly men 65 years and above | 320 | 345 | 410 | 480 | 500 | 40 |
| elderly women 65 years and above | 290 | 320 | 395 | 470 | 500 | 45 |
| boys 3–4 year olds | | 175 | 200 | 220 | | 13 |
| boys 5–7 year olds | | 185 | 215 | 250 | | 20 |
| boys 8–11 year olds | | 205 | 250 | 295 | | 28 |
| boys 12–14 year olds | | 240 | 290 | 340 | | 30 |
| boys 15–18 year olds | | 290 | 330 | 375 | | 26 |
| girls 3–4 year olds | | 175 | 200 | 225 | | 15 |
| girls 5–7 year olds | | 185 | 220 | 260 | | 22 |
| girls 8–11 year olds | | 210 | 260 | 315 | | 32 |
| girls 12–14 year olds | | 260 | 315 | 370 | | 34 |
| girls 15–18 year olds | | 300 | 345 | 385 | | 27 |

| 23. Abdominal depth | 1st %-le | 5th%-le | 50th %-le | 95th%-le | 99th%-le | SD |
|---|---|---|---|---|---|---|
| men aged 19 to 65 years | 185 | 210 | 270 | 330 | 350 | 36 |
| women aged 19 to 65 years | 165 | 190 | 250 | 315 | 340 | 38 |
| male students | 200 | 220 | 275 | 325 | 350 | 32 |
| female students | 170 | 195 | 255 | 320 | 345 | 38 |
| elderly men 65 years and above | 245 | 275 | 340 | 410 | 435 | 40 |
| elderly women 65 years and above | 220 | 250 | 325 | 400 | 430 | 45 |
| boys 3–4 year olds | | 135 | 155 | 170 | | 10 |
| boys 5–7 year olds | | 135 | 160 | 185 | | 16 |
| boys 8–11 year olds | | 145 | 180 | 220 | | 24 |
| boys 12–14 year olds | | 165 | 205 | 245 | | 24 |
| boys 15–18 year olds | | 190 | 230 | 270 | | 25 |
| girls 3–4 year olds | | 135 | 155 | 170 | | 12 |
| girls 5–7 year olds | | 135 | 165 | 195 | | 19 |
| girls 8–11 year olds | | 145 | 190 | 230 | | 27 |
| girls 12–14 year olds | | 165 | 210 | 250 | | 25 |
| girls 15–18 year olds | | 185 | 220 | 255 | | 21 |

| 24. Chest depth | 1st %-le | 5th%-le | 50th %-le | 95th%-le | 99th%-le | SD |
|---|---|---|---|---|---|---|
| men aged 19 to 65 years | 190 | 205 | 245 | 290 | 305 | 25 |
| women aged 19 to 65 years | 175 | 195 | 250 | 300 | 325 | 32 |
| male students | 200 | 215 | 250 | 290 | 305 | 22 |
| female students | 180 | 205 | 255 | 310 | 330 | 32 |
| elderly men 65 years and above | 170 | 190 | 235 | 280 | 295 | 27 |
| elderly women 65 years and above | 240 | 265 | 325 | 390 | 410 | 37 |
| boys 3–4 year olds | | 105 | 130 | 150 | | 12 |
| boys 5–7 year olds | | 110 | 140 | 170 | | 18 |
| boys 8–11 year olds | | 120 | 160 | 200 | | 24 |
| boys 12–14 year olds | | 140 | 185 | 230 | | 29 |
| boys 15–18 year olds | | 170 | 220 | 265 | | 28 |
| girls 3–4 year olds | | 105 | 125 | 150 | | 13 |
| girls 5–7 year olds | | 110 | 140 | 170 | | 18 |
| girls 8–11 year olds | | 110 | 160 | 210 | | 30 |
| girls 12–14 year olds | | 145 | 200 | 250 | | 31 |
| girls 15–18 year olds | | 185 | 225 | 265 | | 26 |

| 25. Span | 1st %-le | 5th%-le | 50th %-le | 95th%-le | 99th%-le | SD |
|---|---|---|---|---|---|---|
| men aged 19 to 65 years | 1585 | 1645 | 1785 | 1925 | 1980 | 85 |
| women aged 19 to 65 years | 1400 | 1460 | 1595 | 1730 | 1790 | 83 |
| male students | 1640 | 1695 | 1815 | 1940 | 1995 | 76 |
| female students | 1440 | 1495 | 1635 | 1775 | 1830 | 84 |
| elderly men 65 years and above | 1465 | 1530 | 1685 | 1840 | 1900 | 94 |
| elderly women 65 years and above | 1285 | 1345 | 1500 | 1655 | 1720 | 94 |
| boys 3–4 year olds | | 905 | 1010 | 1110 | | 63 |
| boys 5–7 year olds | | 1020 | 1160 | 1300 | | 85 |
| boys 8–11 year olds | | 1205 | 1360 | 1520 | | 96 |
| boys 12–14 year olds | | 1380 | 1585 | 1790 | | 125 |
| boys 15–18 year olds | | 1630 | 1785 | 1935 | | 92 |
| girls 3–4 year olds | | 860 | 980 | 1095 | | 70 |
| girls 5–7 year olds | | 985 | 1125 | 1265 | | 85 |
| girls 8–11 year olds | | 1170 | 1335 | 1495 | | 98 |
| girls 12–14 year olds | | 1370 | 1535 | 1695 | | 99 |
| girls 15–18 year olds | | 1505 | 1610 | 1720 | | 65 |

| 26. Elbow span | 1st %-le | 5th%-le | 50th %-le | 95th%-le | 99th%-le | SD |
|---|---|---|---|---|---|---|
| men aged 19 to 65 years | 845 | 880 | 960 | 1040 | 1075 | 49 |
| women aged 19 to 65 years | 785 | 815 | 890 | 960 | 990 | 44 |
| male students | 875 | 905 | 980 | 1050 | 1080 | 44 |
| female students | 805 | 835 | 910 | 985 | 1015 | 44 |
| elderly men 65 years and above | 780 | 815 | 905 | 995 | 1030 | 54 |
| elderly women 65 years and above | 720 | 755 | 835 | 915 | 950 | 49 |
| boys 3–4 year olds | | 475 | 530 | 590 | | 35 |
| boys 5–7 year olds | | 535 | 610 | 690 | | 47 |
| boys 8–11 year olds | | 630 | 720 | 805 | | 53 |
| boys 12–14 year olds | | 720 | 835 | 950 | | 69 |
| boys 15–18 year olds | | 855 | 940 | 1025 | | 52 |
| girls 3–4 year olds | | 450 | 515 | 585 | | 41 |
| girls 5–7 year olds | | 515 | 595 | 675 | | 49 |
| girls 8–11 year olds | | 610 | 705 | 795 | | 56 |
| girls 12–14 year olds | | 715 | 810 | 905 | | 58 |
| girls 15–18 year olds | | 785 | 850 | 915 | | 40 |

| 27. Standing vertical reach | 1st %-le | 5th%-le | 50th %-le | 95th%-le | 99th%-le | SD |
|---|---|---|---|---|---|---|
| men aged 19 to 65 years | 1975 | 2040 | 2195 | 2350 | 2410 | 94 |
| women aged 19 to 65 years | 1815 | 1880 | 2030 | 2180 | 2245 | 92 |
| male students | 2040 | 2100 | 2235 | 2370 | 2430 | 83 |
| female students | 1865 | 1930 | 2080 | 2235 | 2300 | 93 |
| elderly men 65 years and above | 1730 | 1800 | 1970 | 2140 | 2210 | 104 |
| elderly women 65 years and above | 1560 | 1640 | 1820 | 2005 | 2110 | 112 |
| boys 3–4 year olds | | 1030 | 1175 | 1315 | | 85 |
| boys 5–7 year olds | | 1215 | 1390 | 1565 | | 108 |
| boys 8–11 year olds | | 1460 | 1645 | 1830 | | 112 |
| boys 12–14 year olds | | 1705 | 1910 | 2115 | | 125 |
| boys 15–18 year olds | | 1955 | 2110 | 2260 | | 93 |
| girls 3–4 year olds | | 1035 | 1165 | 1295 | | 78 |
| girls 5–7 year olds | | 1210 | 1375 | 1540 | | 101 |
| girls 8–11 year olds | | 1440 | 1655 | 1865 | | 129 |
| girls 12–14 year olds | | 1695 | 1885 | 2075 | | 116 |
| girls 15–18 year olds | | 1825 | 1965 | 2110 | | 87 |

| 28. Sitting vertical reach | 1st %-le | 5th%-le | 50th %-le | 95th%-le | 99th%-le | SD |
|---|---|---|---|---|---|---|
| men aged 19 to 65 years | 1225 | 1265 | 1360 | 1460 | 1500 | 59 |
| women aged 19 to 65 years | 1135 | 1170 | 1260 | 1345 | 1380 | 53 |
| male students | 1265 | 1300 | 1385 | 1475 | 1510 | 53 |
| female students | 1165 | 1205 | 1290 | 1380 | 1415 | 53 |
| elderly men 65 years and above | 1095 | 1135 | 1240 | 1345 | 1390 | 65 |
| elderly women 65 years and above | 990 | 1035 | 1150 | 1265 | 1315 | 70 |
| boys 3–4 year olds | | 650 | 720 | 795 | | 44 |
| boys 5–7 year olds | | 715 | 810 | 905 | | 57 |
| boys 8–11 year olds | | 830 | 940 | 1045 | | 65 |
| boys 12–14 year olds | | 945 | 1085 | 1225 | | 86 |
| boys 15–18 year olds | | 1120 | 1225 | 1330 | | 64 |
| girls 3–4 year olds | | 620 | 700 | 780 | | 49 |
| girls 5–7 year olds | | 700 | 790 | 885 | | 56 |
| girls 8–11 year olds | | 810 | 925 | 1040 | | 70 |
| girls 12–14 year olds | | 940 | 1070 | 1205 | | 80 |
| girls 15–18 year olds | | 1035 | 1135 | 1235 | | 61 |

| 29. Horizontal forward reach | 1st %-le | 5th%-le | 50th %-le | 95th%-le | 99th%-le | SD |
|---|---|---|---|---|---|---|
| men aged 19 to 65 years | 685 | 715 | 780 | 850 | 880 | 41 |
| women aged 19 to 65 years | 640 | 665 | 725 | 785 | 810 | 37 |
| male students | 710 | 735 | 795 | 855 | 880 | 37 |
| female students | 655 | 680 | 740 | 805 | 830 | 37 |
| elderly men 65 years and above | 635 | 665 | 740 | 815 | 845 | 45 |
| elderly women 65 years and above | 585 | 615 | 680 | 750 | 775 | 41 |
| boys 3–4 year olds | | 370 | 430 | 490 | | 36 |
| boys 5–7 year olds | | 430 | 495 | 560 | | 38 |
| boys 8–11 year olds | | 495 | 565 | 635 | | 42 |
| boys 12–14 year olds | | 570 | 650 | 735 | | 50 |
| boys 15–18 year olds | | 650 | 725 | 795 | | 45 |
| girls 3–4 year olds | | 365 | 430 | 495 | | 40 |
| girls 5–7 year olds | | 420 | 485 | 545 | | 37 |
| girls 8–11 year olds | | 490 | 570 | 645 | | 48 |
| girls 12–14 year olds | | 570 | 640 | 710 | | 43 |
| girls 15–18 year olds | | 605 | 670 | 730 | | 39 |

| 30. Elbow finger tip length | 1st %-le | 5th%-le | 50th %-le | 95th%-le | 99th%-le | SD |
|---|---|---|---|---|---|---|
| men aged 19 to 65 years | 415 | 430 | 470 | 510 | 525 | 24 |
| women aged 19 to 65 years | 390 | 405 | 440 | 475 | 490 | 21 |
| male students | 430 | 445 | 480 | 515 | 530 | 21 |
| female students | 400 | 415 | 450 | 485 | 500 | 21 |
| elderly men 65 years and above | 385 | 400 | 445 | 490 | 505 | 26 |
| elderly women 65 years and above | 360 | 375 | 415 | 450 | 470 | 24 |
| boys 3–4 year olds | | 240 | 270 | 295 | | 17 |
| boys 5–7 year olds | | 275 | 310 | 345 | | 23 |
| boys 8–11 year olds | | 320 | 365 | 405 | | 27 |
| boys 12–14 year olds | | 365 | 420 | 475 | | 33 |
| boys 15–18 year olds | | 435 | 470 | 510 | | 23 |
| girls 3–4 year olds | | 235 | 265 | 295 | | 20 |
| girls 5–7 year olds | | 270 | 305 | 340 | | 22 |
| girls 8–11 year olds | | 310 | 360 | 410 | | 31 |
| girls 12–14 year olds | | 370 | 410 | 450 | | 25 |
| girls 15–18 year olds | | 395 | 425 | 455 | | 17 |

| 31. Acromion grip length | 1st %-le | 5th%-le | 50th %-le | 95th%-le | 99th%-le | SD |
|---|---|---|---|---|---|---|
| men aged 19 to 65 years | 555 | 580 | 640 | 695 | 720 | 36 |
| women aged 19 to 65 years | 515 | 540 | 590 | 640 | 665 | 31 |
| male students | 575 | 600 | 650 | 700 | 725 | 31 |
| female students | 530 | 555 | 605 | 660 | 680 | 32 |
| elderly men 65 years and above | 510 | 540 | 600 | 665 | 695 | 39 |
| elderly women 65 years and above | 475 | 495 | 555 | 615 | 640 | 36 |
| boys 3–4 year olds | | 325 | 375 | 420 | | 29 |
| boys 5–7 year olds | | 365 | 425 | 490 | | 37 |
| boys 8–11 year olds | | 430 | 500 | 570 | | 43 |
| boys 12–14 year olds | | 500 | 585 | 670 | | 51 |
| boys 15–18 year olds | | 600 | 665 | 730 | | 40 |
| girls 3–4 year olds | | 300 | 360 | 415 | | 36 |
| girls 5–7 year olds | | 350 | 415 | 480 | | 40 |
| girls 8–11 year olds | | 410 | 490 | 570 | | 49 |
| girls 12–14 year olds | | 490 | 570 | 650 | | 48 |
| girls 15–18 year olds | | 545 | 595 | 645 | | 30 |

| 32. Foot length | 1st %-le | 5th%-le | 50th %-le | 95th%-le | 99th%-le | SD |
|---|---|---|---|---|---|---|
| men aged 19 to 65 years | 235 | 245 | 265 | 290 | 300 | 14 |
| women aged 19 to 65 years | 210 | 220 | 240 | 255 | 265 | 12 |
| male students | 245 | 250 | 270 | 290 | 300 | 12 |
| female students | 215 | 225 | 245 | 265 | 270 | 12 |
| elderly men 65 years and above | 215 | 225 | 250 | 275 | 285 | 15 |
| elderly women 65 years and above | 195 | 200 | 225 | 245 | 255 | 13 |
| boys 3–4 year olds | | 140 | 160 | 180 | | 11 |
| boys 5–7 year olds | | 160 | 185 | 210 | | 14 |
| boys 8–11 year olds | | 185 | 215 | 240 | | 16 |
| boys 12–14 year olds | | 215 | 245 | 275 | | 17 |
| boys 15–18 year olds | | 240 | 265 | 285 | | 14 |
| girls 3–4 year olds | | 140 | 160 | 180 | | 12 |
| girls 5–7 year olds | | 155 | 180 | 205 | | 14 |
| girls 8–11 year olds | | 185 | 210 | 235 | | 15 |
| girls 12–14 year olds | | 210 | 230 | 255 | | 13 |
| girls 15–18 year olds | | 220 | 240 | 260 | | 12 |

| 33. Heel ball length | 1st %-le | 5th%-le | 50th %-le | 95th%-le | 99th%-le | SD |
|---|---|---|---|---|---|---|
| men aged 19 to 65 years | 170 | 175 | 195 | 210 | 220 | 11 |
| women aged 19 to 65 years | 150 | 160 | 170 | 185 | 190 | 9 |
| male students | 175 | 185 | 200 | 215 | 220 | 9 |
| female students | 155 | 160 | 175 | 190 | 195 | 9 |
| elderly men 65 years and above | 155 | 165 | 185 | 205 | 210 | 12 |
| elderly women 65 years and above | 140 | 145 | 160 | 180 | 185 | 10 |

| 34. Foot breadth | 1st %-le | 5th%-le | 50th %-le | 95th%-le | 99th%-le | SD |
|---|---|---|---|---|---|---|
| men aged 19 to 65 years | 85 | 90 | 100 | 110 | 115 | 6 |
| women aged 19 to 65 years | 75 | 80 | 90 | 100 | 105 | 6 |
| male students | 90 | 95 | 105 | 110 | 115 | 6 |
| female students | 80 | 85 | 90 | 100 | 105 | 6 |
| elderly men 65 years and above | 80 | 85 | 95 | 105 | 110 | 7 |
| elderly women 65 years and above | 70 | 75 | 85 | 95 | 100 | 6 |
| boys 3–4 year olds | | 60 | 65 | 70 | | 4 |
| boys 5–7 year olds | | 65 | 75 | 85 | | 6 |
| boys 8–11 year olds | | 70 | 85 | 95 | | 6 |
| boys 12–14 year olds | | 80 | 90 | 105 | | 7 |
| boys 15–18 year olds | | 90 | 100 | 110 | | 6 |
| girls 3–4 year olds | | 55 | 65 | 70 | | 5 |
| girls 5–7 year olds | | 60 | 70 | 80 | | 6 |
| girls 8–11 year olds | | 70 | 80 | 90 | | 7 |
| girls 12–14 year olds | | 75 | 90 | 100 | | 7 |
| girls 15–18 year olds | | 80 | 90 | 100 | | 5 |

| 35. Ankle height | 1st %-le | 5th%-le | 50th %-le | 95th%-le | 99th%-le | SD |
|---|---|---|---|---|---|---|
| men aged 19 to 65 years | 55 | 60 | 75 | 85 | 90 | 7 |
| women aged 19 to 65 years | 55 | 60 | 70 | 75 | 80 | 6 |
| male students | 60 | 65 | 75 | 85 | 90 | 6 |
| female students | 55 | 60 | 70 | 80 | 85 | 6 |
| elderly men 65 years and above | 50 | 55 | 70 | 80 | 85 | 7 |
| elderly women 65 years and above | 50 | 50 | 65 | 75 | 80 | 7 |

| 36. Hand length | 1st %-le | 5th%-le | 50th %-le | 95th%-le | 99th%-le | SD |
|---|---|---|---|---|---|---|
| men aged 19 to 65 years | 165 | 175 | 190 | 205 | 215 | 10 |
| women aged 19 to 65 years | 150 | 155 | 170 | 185 | 190 | 9 |
| male students | 170 | 180 | 195 | 210 | 215 | 9 |
| female students | 155 | 160 | 175 | 190 | 195 | 9 |
| elderly men 65 years and above | 155 | 160 | 180 | 195 | 205 | 11 |
| elderly women 65 years and above | 135 | 145 | 160 | 175 | 185 | 10 |
| boys 3–4 year olds | | 100 | 115 | 125 | | 8 |
| boys 5–7 year olds | | 115 | 130 | 145 | | 10 |
| boys 8–11 year olds | | 130 | 150 | 165 | | 11 |
| boys 12–14 year olds | | 150 | 170 | 195 | | 13 |
| boys 15–18 year olds | | 170 | 190 | 205 | | 9 |
| girls 3–4 year olds | | 100 | 115 | 130 | | 9 |
| girls 5–7 year olds | | 110 | 125 | 145 | | 10 |
| girls 8–11 year olds | | 130 | 150 | 165 | | 11 |
| girls 12–14 year olds | | 150 | 170 | 185 | | 10 |
| girls 15–18 year olds | | 160 | 175 | 190 | | 9 |

| 37. Hand breadth (metacarpal) | 1st %-le | 5th%-le | 50th %-le | 95th%-le | 99th%-le | SD |
|---|---|---|---|---|---|---|
| men aged 19 to 65 years | 75 | 80 | 90 | 95 | 100 | 5 |
| women aged 19 to 65 years | 65 | 70 | 75 | 85 | 85 | 5 |
| male students | 80 | 85 | 90 | 100 | 100 | 5 |
| female students | 65 | 70 | 80 | 85 | 90 | 5 |
| elderly men 65 years and above | 70 | 75 | 85 | 95 | 95 | 6 |
| elderly women 65 years and above | 60 | 60 | 70 | 80 | 85 | 5 |
| boys 3–4 year olds | | 50 | 55 | 60 | | 4 |
| boys 5–7 year olds | | 55 | 60 | 70 | | 5 |
| boys 8–11 year olds | | 60 | 70 | 75 | | 5 |
| boys 12–14 year olds | | 70 | 80 | 90 | | 7 |
| boys 15–18 year olds | | 80 | 90 | 95 | | 5 |
| girls 3–4 year olds | | 45 | 55 | 60 | | 5 |
| girls 5–7 year olds | | 50 | 60 | 65 | | 5 |
| girls 8–11 year olds | | 60 | 70 | 75 | | 5 |
| girls 12–14 year olds | | 65 | 75 | 80 | | 5 |
| girls 15–18 year olds | | 70 | 75 | 80 | | 4 |

| 38. Head depth | 1st %-le | 5th%-le | 50th %-le | 95th%-le | 99th%-le | SD |
|---|---|---|---|---|---|---|
| men aged 19 to 65 years | 180 | 185 | 195 | 205 | 210 | 7 |
| women aged 19 to 65 years | 165 | 170 | 185 | 195 | 200 | 7 |
| male students | 185 | 190 | 200 | 210 | 215 | 6 |
| female students | 170 | 175 | 190 | 200 | 205 | 7 |
| elderly men 65 years and above | 165 | 170 | 185 | 195 | 200 | 8 |
| elderly women 65 years and above | 155 | 160 | 170 | 185 | 190 | 8 |
| boys 3–4 year olds | | 170 | 180 | 190 | | 7 |
| boys 5–7 year olds | | 165 | 180 | 195 | | 9 |
| boys 8–11 year olds | | 165 | 185 | 205 | | 11 |
| boys 12–14 year olds | | 170 | 190 | 205 | | 11 |
| boys 15–18 year olds | | 185 | 200 | 210 | | 8 |
| girls 3–4 year olds | | 155 | 165 | 175 | | 7 |
| girls 5–7 year olds | | 155 | 170 | 180 | | 7 |
| girls 8–11 year olds | | 155 | 175 | 190 | | 11 |
| girls 12–14 year olds | | 160 | 175 | 190 | | 9 |
| girls 15–18 year olds | | 170 | 180 | 190 | | 8 |

| 39. Head breadth | 1st %-le | 5th%-le | 50th %-le | 95th%-le | 99th%-le | SD |
|---|---|---|---|---|---|---|
| men aged 19 to 65 years | 140 | 145 | 155 | 165 | 170 | 6 |
| women aged 19 to 65 years | 130 | 135 | 145 | 150 | 155 | 6 |
| male students | 145 | 150 | 160 | 165 | 170 | 6 |
| female students | 135 | 135 | 145 | 155 | 160 | 6 |
| elderly men 65 years and above | 130 | 135 | 145 | 160 | 160 | 7 |
| elderly women 65 years and above | 120 | 125 | 135 | 145 | 150 | 6 |
| boys 3–4 year olds | | 130 | 140 | 150 | | 6 |
| boys 5–7 year olds | | 130 | 140 | 150 | | 5 |
| boys 8–11 year olds | | 130 | 145 | 160 | | 9 |
| boys 12–14 year olds | | 135 | 150 | 165 | | 9 |
| boys 15–18 year olds | | 145 | 155 | 165 | | 6 |
| girls 3–4 year olds | | 120 | 130 | 140 | | 6 |
| girls 5–7 year olds | | 125 | 135 | 145 | | 6 |
| girls 8–11 year olds | | 120 | 135 | 150 | | 9 |
| girls 12–14 year olds | | 125 | 140 | 155 | | 9 |
| girls 15–18 year olds | | 135 | 145 | 155 | | 5 |

| 40. Slumped sitting height | 1st %-le | 5th%-le | 50th %-le | 95th%-le | 99th%-le | SD |
|---|---|---|---|---|---|---|
| men aged 19 to 65 years | 775 | 800 | 865 | 925 | 950 | 38 |
| women aged 19 to 65 years | 720 | 745 | 805 | 860 | 885 | 35 |
| male students | 805 | 825 | 880 | 935 | 960 | 33 |
| female students | 740 | 765 | 825 | 885 | 910 | 36 |

| 41. Slumped sitting eye height | 1st %-le | 5th%-le | 50th %-le | 95th%-le | 99th%-le | SD |
|---|---|---|---|---|---|---|
| men aged 19 to 65 years | 670 | 695 | 760 | 825 | 850 | 39 |
| women aged 19 to 65 years | 625 | 645 | 700 | 755 | 775 | 33 |
| male students | 695 | 720 | 775 | 830 | 855 | 34 |
| female students | 640 | 665 | 720 | 775 | 795 | 33 |

| 42. Slumped sitting shoulder height | 1st %-le | 5th%-le | 50th %-le | 95th%-le | 99th%-le | SD |
|---|---|---|---|---|---|---|
| men aged 19 to 65 years | 490 | 510 | 570 | 630 | 655 | 35 |
| women aged 19 to 65 years | 460 | 480 | 535 | 590 | 610 | 33 |
| male students | 510 | 530 | 580 | 635 | 655 | 31 |
| female students | 470 | 495 | 550 | 605 | 625 | 33 |

| 43. Elbow vertical distance | 1st %-le | 5th%-le | 50th %-le | 95th%-le | 99th%-le | SD |
|---|---|---|---|---|---|---|
| men aged 19 to 65 years | 475 | 500 | 560 | 625 | 650 | 38 |
| women aged 19 to 65 years | 435 | 460 | 510 | 565 | 585 | 32 |
| male students | 495 | 515 | 570 | 630 | 650 | 34 |
| female students | 450 | 470 | 525 | 580 | 600 | 32 |

| 44. Fingertip eye horizontal distance | 1st %-le | 5th%-le | 50th %-le | 95th%-le | 99th%-le | SD |
|---|---|---|---|---|---|---|
| men aged 19 to 65 years | 330 | 345 | 375 | 405 | 415 | 19 |
| women aged 19 to 65 years | 310 | 320 | 345 | 375 | 385 | 17 |
| male students | 340 | 355 | 380 | 410 | 420 | 17 |
| female students | 315 | 330 | 355 | 385 | 395 | 17 |

| 45. Elbow rest height minus thigh clearance | 1st %-le | 5th%-le | 50th %-le | 95th%-le | 99th%-le | SD |
|---|---|---|---|---|---|---|
| men aged 19 to 65 years | 30 | 45 | 85 | 130 | 145 | 25 |
| women aged 19 to 65 years | 25 | 45 | 90 | 130 | 150 | 27 |
| male students | 35 | 50 | 90 | 125 | 140 | 23 |
| female students | 25 | 45 | 90 | 135 | 155 | 27 |

| 46. Buttock knee length minus abdominal depth | 1st %-le | 5th%-le | 50th %-le | 95th%-le | 99th%-le | SD |
|---|---|---|---|---|---|---|
| men aged 19 to 65 years | 220 | 250 | 325 | 400 | 430 | 46 |
| women aged 19 to 65 years | 230 | 255 | 320 | 385 | 410 | 40 |
| male students | 235 | 265 | 330 | 400 | 425 | 41 |
| female students | 235 | 260 | 330 | 395 | 420 | 40 |

| 47. Elbow fingertip length minus abdominal depth | 1st %-le | 5th%-le | 50th %-le | 95th%-le | 99th%-le | SD |
|---|---|---|---|---|---|---|
| men aged 19 to 65 years | 100 | 130 | 205 | 275 | 305 | 44 |
| women aged 19 to 65 years | 55 | 95 | 190 | 285 | 320 | 57 |
| male students | 115 | 145 | 205 | 270 | 295 | 39 |
| female students | 55 | 95 | 195 | 290 | 330 | 58 |

| 48. Horizontal forward reach minus abdominal depth | 1st %-le | 5th%-le | 50th %-le | 95th%-le | 99th%-le | SD |
|---|---|---|---|---|---|---|
| men aged 19 to 65 years | 415 | 445 | 515 | 585 | 610 | 42 |
| women aged 19 to 65 years | 350 | 385 | 475 | 560 | 595 | 53 |
| male students | 440 | 465 | 525 | 585 | 610 | 37 |
| female students | 360 | 395 | 485 | 575 | 610 | 53 |

| 49. Standard seat height plus elbow rest height | 1st %-le | 5th%-le | 50th %-le | 95th%-le | 99th%-le | SD |
|---|---|---|---|---|---|---|
| men aged 19 to 65 years | 560 | 585 | 650 | 715 | 745 | 39 |
| women aged 19 to 65 years | 525 | 550 | 605 | 660 | 685 | 34 |
| male students | 585 | 605 | 665 | 720 | 745 | 35 |
| female students | 540 | 565 | 620 | 680 | 700 | 35 |

| 50. Standard seat height plus thigh clearance | 1st %-le | 5th%-le | 50th %-le | 95th%-le | 99th%-le | SD |
|---|---|---|---|---|---|---|
| men aged 19 to 65 years | 465 | 495 | 565 | 635 | 665 | 42 |
| women aged 19 to 65 years | 445 | 465 | 520 | 570 | 590 | 32 |
| male students | 490 | 515 | 575 | 635 | 660 | 37 |
| female students | 455 | 480 | 530 | 585 | 605 | 32 |

# Index